CRACKING THE CHRONIC ILLNESS CODE

For a FASTER healing 90-DAY PROGRAM

KARRIE WILSON

ISBN
978-1-958690-14-7 (Paperback)
978-1-958690-15-4 (eBook)
978-1-958690-13-0 (Hardcover)

DEDICATION

To my daughter Barissa:

Because of your love and faith, I have healed and have the best gift of all—that is, being your mother. I could never ask for a better daughter than you.

ACKNOWLEDGEMENTS

Mother:

    At the end of the day, it's about who you`ve lifted, who you made better, and what you`ve given back. Your heart is pure as gold, and there are very few left in this world who care as much as you do. You help me understand myself in a world that is constantly trying to make me something else. Thank you for truly believing that I could and making this book happen.

TABLE OF CONTENTS

HUMAN BODY

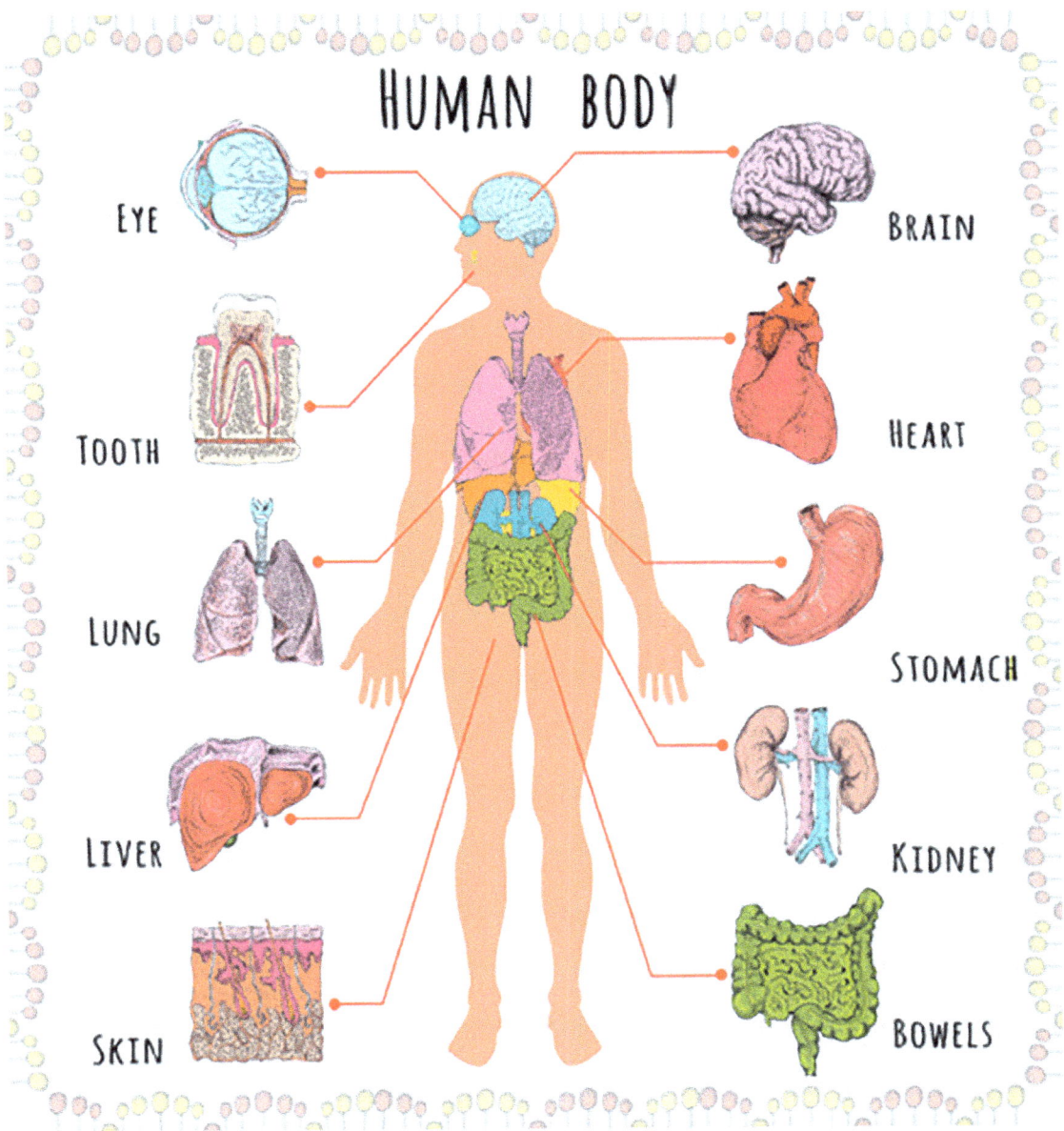

EYE

BRAIN

TOOTH

HEART

LUNG

STOMACH

LIVER

KIDNEY

SKIN

BOWELS

INTRODUCTION

I walked into my doctor's office knowing I was going to hear the same thing again. "More drugs, scans, surgery and put a colostrum bag on me." The only thing I could think of was holding back the tears in my eyes and explaining to my daughter why this bag was attached to me. My confidence just flew out the window and took my love life with it. Not only am I going to have pain still, but I also have a bag attached to me.

As the doctor kept talking, All I could think was why is he making this choice and not me? Everything in your life is a choice you have made, and if you want a different result, you make a different choice. I looked up, and I did something I had never done before. I told the doctor no! I am done with all the medications and surgeries. I want to fix myself naturally without surgery. He then proceeded to tell me the same thing again "If you get off the medicine, then you will be permanently damaged or might even die." He was not willing to go any other way except for the surgery. Many other doctors told me the same. I just got up and left. I don't know if I was still in shock because I kept thinking maybe I was wrong and I should turn back. But at that moment, I realized that the decision you make could change the course of your life forever.

My name is Karrie Wilson, and I have broken The Chronic Illness Code for my Crohns. I am here to help you see a different way of looking at your illness. To show you how I walked the path of me curing my chronic illness and how I kicked the habit of medication and got rid of my Crohns when surgery was not an option for me. I am health coach certified as well as a chronic illness coach. I have taken many classes on diseases and disorders.

I was devastated when I got diagnosed with Crohn's! Which caused me to have many problems. I wasn't able to keep food down properly, and pain throughout my body all the time. I was in and out of the hospital almost every month, doctor's appointments every other day, and living a life as if I was an older lady. It was so overwhelming to find the right information. I was getting a lot of wrong information from doctors as they were trying to figure it out. I had to figure something out or live like this forever.

I had to get off all this medication. I had read that the medication Cipro (Ciprofloxacin) that was the antibiotics I was taking, had an ongoing lawsuit against them. The medication has been linked to a severe form of nerve damage called peripheral neuropathy, tendon ruptures, and aortic aneurysm. It belongs to a class of drugs called Fluoroquinolones, which fight bacterial infections of the skin, urinary infection, and gastrointestinal system—manufactured by Bayer, which we all know as the company that makes headache medicine. That also paid for not letting food industries spend tons of money on labeling what is in our food. Cipro was approved by the U.s Food & Drug Administration (FDA) in 1987 and still is being used. People with this disease may experience tingling, numbness, unusual sensations, weakness, or burning pain in the affected areas. In most patients, symptoms are symmetrical, involving both hands and feet.

Here are some signs for symptoms:

- Pain
- Burning
- Tingling
- Numbness
- Change in sensation to light touch, pain, or temperature.
- Change of sense of body position.
- Loss of reflexes.
- Paresthesia
- Muscle wasting
- Paralysis

Early diagnosis is important because nerves have a limited capacity to regenerate, and treatment may only slow the progression of the disease. If the patient is severely impaired, they may need physical therapy to help regain their strength and avoid muscle cramping and/or spasms.

People will still use this medication as it does help very quickly for bacterial infections and UTIs. Using them for a short time may or may not hurt you. People with Crohn's and other autoimmune disorders are told to take this usually three times a day until they go into remission or until they find a better drug.

Here are some signs of side effects:

- Permanent nerve damage
- Tendon ruptures
- Central nervous system disorders
- Tremors
- Confusion
- Loss of consciousness
- Cardiovascular collapse
- Life-threatening skin reactions

In 2003, a group of U.S. postal workers filed a Cipro lawsuit against Bayer. They were prescribed Cipro during the 2001 anthrax scare and shortly after that began experiencing severe side effects. The complaint stated that Bayer failed to disclose information regarding the drug's potential to cause nerve and tendon damage, as well as other serious injuries. Now in 2016, for the second time, the FDA has upgraded warnings on this antibiotic drug, saying they're too strong to be used for sinus infections, bronchitis, and urinary tract infections. They're causing disabling side effects and advised to stop using them. Adverse reactions can occur immediately from as little as one pill, within weeks, months, or even longer after stopping them. You can read more about this at Quinolone Vigilance Foundation. I also had doctors having me sign contracts letting me know that some of these medications could eventually give me cancer by using them longer than two years.

These kinds of things scared me as the pain in my fingers started to get worse.

No one will give me the right answers now, and I had to take matters into my own hands. If I wanted to do it right, I had to do it myself. I started to read as much as I could. I started learning anything about the biology of humans, diseases and disorders, and pain management. I needed to start from the beginning. Once I understood that my goal was to get off all medications, I started reading a few books like:

1. **Mastering The Zone, Barry Sears, Ph.D.**
2. **Meditation to heal the depression and your mind**
3. **Jini Patel Thompson, Ph.D. "Listen to Your Gut"**

4. **Kevin Trudeau, Natural cures They Don`t Want You to Know About.**
5. **Dr. Alice Robert, The complete human body.**
6. **Steven R. Gundry, The Plant Paradox**
7. **The Complete Human Body by Dr. Alice Roberts**

Human Biology is a study that examines humans through genetics, evolution, physiology, anatomy, epidemiology, anthropology, ecology, nutrition, population genetics, and sociocultural influences. This is where I believe where you can find answers to curing yourself. You can`t just consider one part; it needs to be the whole thing to study, and then you can get an idea of where to start to heal.

While I was finding my healing, I decided to get some certificates/ classes like:

- Nutrition, Chronic Disease and Health certificate
- Health coach certificate
- Classes on disease and disorders
- Bacteriology, anatomy, and physiology
- Infection Control/chemistry
- Medical Terminology/Billing and Coding
- Chemical procedures/practices
- Anatomy of skin/Body system/Cells/Tissue
- Relaxation treatments/Electricity principles/safety

I learned quickly through my pain and eagerness to get rid of it as doctors could only prescribe me dangerous anti-inflammatory medication or cut out tissue. The pain killers were opium's that knocked me out. The antibiotics had a lawsuit against them because it was causing permanent joint damage, which I didn't want.

Experience is the best teacher you will learn more from, things that happen to you in real life than you would from hearing about or studying. I would never want a person to go through what I did. Yet there're many of them living with chronic conditions like it's a normal part of life. I wanted those suffering from chronic illness to seek knowledge through me or realize there is another way to not deal with the pain.

All the information was confusing at first, but I got it all in order and am ready to share it with you. I am a very visual person, and science was not easy. I had to put it in a way I understood it visually.

I wanted to write this book to show you visually, step by step, to take from the beginning to the end. I noticed many people, including me, would be hesitant to start or just give up too easily. I needed a kick in the butt sometimes. Having coaches keeps you motivated; you will get the correct information and get healed a lot faster than by yourself. We have parts inside our bodies that need to be taken care of that you didn't know you had to repair—from a person who has been through the same path would help you achieve this.

You wouldn't have to play scavenger hunt to break the chronic code. I also wanted to show you how I got off my medication, repaired my body, and did it naturally without surgery; by understanding what was inside my body and why it was so important to fix it.

I do believe that I have helped my disorder and have been in remission for over 17 years. I am doing things that I have not been able to do in a long time, as I can now eat food without the pain and throwing up. I can be a regular person again and feel the best I have ever felt in my life.

As you develop your personalized program just for your chronic conditions, I promise you it will be easy. Make sure you know how it's healing you and why. It would be best if you kept goals and food diaries. Give yourself two weeks and write down how your body feels. If you feel sicker, then switch your diet. You will get started on the first day, knowing better knowledge of your condition and how to relieve the pain to relax and start the healing process. You need a professional to show you what you need and for how long as I work with a team consisting of naturopathic doctors, nutritionists, herbalists, mineralogists, toxicologists, medical doctors, and microbiologists. We work as a team to make sure you get all the correct information. Some of the natural stuff I use is amazing but, at the same time, is very strong and can burn your skin.

Minerals are important for your body to stay healthy. Your body uses minerals to keep your bones, muscles, heart, and brain working properly. It will make enzymes and hormones. Some minerals like DMSO will pull things through your skin like lotion being left on your hands and it will pull through your blood stream and you can taste it on your tongue in seconds. It will be very dangerous if you use it wrong, but that stuff is amazing in healing you. Your skin has pores that open and absorb anything you rub on it. We have minerals that pull plaque off your teeth. It will build strong enamel on them to make them stronger and white. It has a pulling effect on it. It can help cleanse your body. It's called Bentonite clay. A lot of this stuff is kept hidden from us for their personal gain. But these amazing tools were given to us to heal us. We need the knowledge of these powerful tools.

I can introduce some of these items that you never knew existed to help you heal through your journey.

Here are some ways that I can help you through your journey of healing:

- Personalize an eating plan just for your body type and disorder
- Teach you to look at food differently
- Know if what you`re putting in your mouth is nutritional.
- Sunday meal preps for the week. so, you're not having lasting pain, healthier and
- enjoyable meals.
- Are those vitamins needed for your disorder, or if you're wasting your money?
- Help you to really understand the underlining of your pain and disorder.
- know if your body is having a reaction from food or allergies.
- Learn how to cook healthy meals and condiments from home with good ingredients.
- Learn where the healthy fast foods are and what oils they use for cooking their food in.
- Minerals like Baking soda can relieve constipation and alkaline the body when it's mixed with acid in your body.
- Learn what prebiotics, probiotics, and enzymes do for your body.
- Learn meditation from Mindfullness.com and ASMR from YouTube to heal your stress, anxiety and be more confident.
- Learn about Body Mapping and Face Mapping to heal the body.

While 90 days might seem long, it's a very realistic time frame to heal naturally fully. You will see results in as little as a week, but I want you to make enough T-Cells to fight the disease and gain the knowledge. I will be with you through the whole journey, so don't give up. When you have questions or need a coach, you can check out my website at Gutpaincoach.com.

You do not need to leave the house if you're not feeling good. When you are resting, your body is weak, and you need to remember that you're not wasting your day by doing nothing. You're exactly doing what you need to do. You're recovering. Watching someone who has done it before and seeing how they improved is a great way to learn.

The past 17 years of battling Crohn's Disease was the hardest and loneliest time of my life. This disease has taught me how to be my own advocate, understand my body, and give it what it needs to heal, which I have never done before. This journey needed to happen for me to learn all this stuff and get enough passion for helping others. When you wake up every morning fighting the same battle that left you weak the night before, that's bravery, and we all need a helping hand to get through this pain. That's where health coaches come in. We help you implement small changes, little by little, at a pace that's comfortable for you to help you discover your bio-individuality.

Habits don't just happen. It takes 90 days before a new behavior becomes automatic. There is something that will work for you. The trick is finding it in yourself—your easy way. Together we can Crack this Chronic Illness code. Let's get started.

CHAPTER 1

How I learned about my disease and how it changed me forever.

I never cared about learning Biology or how the body works. It never interested me until I was diagnosed with Crohn's. I thought everything I needed to know I learned in school. That wasn't true at all.

Schools were only teaching what everyone would let them teach. The medical industry presents itself as the only source of truth when it comes to health, illness, and disease. They use the words like scientifically tested and scientifically proven. These things they are presenting are only theories and are constantly changing. They told us that removing our tonsils and appendix improved our health, and they told us that butter, eggs, and all alcohol are bad for you, but now it is great for you. It's hard enough for us to decide or come to terms that we need help. We all make mistakes; I understand but let us have the choices to make with our bodies. We don't care until we need to or if it's a dying need. We have too many people that will sue for anything. Doctors are scared to talk about other alternatives. People don't follow directions and do things wrong and blame everyone else. Now we all just put up a blind eye. Then we have the people that want to save money instead of their health.

It's crazy how you try and help people, and they will say; I don't want to hear it, or it costs too much money. I then will watch them in pain and hear them complain about it. I know the result of not taking care of their condition and hope they know too. I know for sure I did my complaining to friends and family. They told me all the time. When you hurt so much, you forget to see the little warning signs your body tells you. You pray so much for it to go away, that you go numb from the pain. You do so much damage to your body and don't realize it. Your body will go into safety mode, and you go numb to the pain, so you don't go into shock. Your body talks to you in a language called SYMPTOMS. If you listen, you will hear it tell you where the problems are.

A few of these symptoms are:

- Headache
- Arm pain
- Digestive issues that keep going
- Dizziness when you move
- Swelling
- Rashes on your body

This will help you with knowing what level of pain you're in. Take notes every day, then add up at the end of two to four weeks.

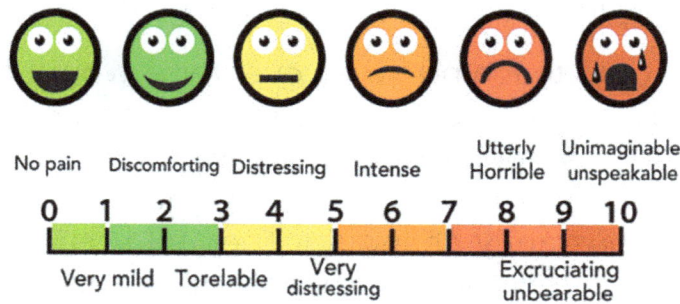

This chart showed me to look at pain differently. When you visually see how many bad days, It will tell you if you have chronic pain or minor pain. Some people have high pain tolerance. Some people don't realize it from always hiding the pain or just getting used to it. This will be a useful tool to monitor your pain and check if you're getting better. We need visual pamphlets to show us what we need to do.

In addition to Crohn's related symptoms, living with a disease may cause feelings of helplessness, isolation and could lead to depression. You isolate yourself at home. The only thing you want to do is sit in the hot bath or sleep to numb the pain. We need not isolate ourselves from other people. We need to get out there and talk to other people with the same problems and learn.

These illnesses could isolate you and make you depressed. Getting out and discovering what you can do for yourself will make big changes. Not knowing what to do can make you believe it's worse than it is.

We also need to learn for ourselves what we need for our health. In this world, we are still primitive creatures, and we will fight for our own lives, not someone else's when it comes down to it. If you want to live, then you need to do this for yourself. While we are healing, it's ok to relax and learn all about what you need.

Here are a few items I loved to use to relax and heal my pain:

- **Epsom Salt -** Drinking it can flush out toxins and relieve constipation.
- **Grey Sea Salt -** Gets rid of mucus from the body and gives you beneficial minerals.
- **Bentonite Clay -** It pulls toxins from within the skin and will give you vitamins and minerals.
- **Oatmeal -** Has avenanthramides which can also reduce inflammation and itching.
- **Baking Soda -** It will neutralize pH level and remove mucus from the body.
- **Meditation -** Help regulate brain activity (Headspace, calm apps).

Constant stress and anxiety will cause illnesses in our bodies and we need to fix them. Repetitive tapping or ASMR is good way to relieve stress or high anxiety.

Different tones also make you not think about the stress you are having at that moment. The tones go from one ear to the other, and your eyes will follow. That's a good way to stop overthinking and calm down. When we go to work and get a lot of stress, we cannot shut it off when we get home. This is the way to help you stop. If you're always hearing negative at your work, then listen to the soothing voice tell you how wonderful you are. You will have tons of confidence after you're done. I know people don't believe that tones or music will heal you. I don't know for sure either, but I know when I had severe anxiety at night, this helped with overthinking everyday stresses. It distracted my thinking when I heard these noises, and that's all I needed to get my sleep. It's like the Tapotement massage technique. Massage therapists use this technique which involves a series of brisk percussions in a rapid, alternating, and rhythmic pattern. It gives the trapped emotional energy (anxiety) a focus and a direction towards release.

What Is an Ecosystem in The Digestive Tract?

There is an ecosystem where 100 trillion bacteria live. Although some bacteria are bad, others are very good. They are crucial for proper digestion. They have important jobs. They help break down food, create some vitamins, work with the immune system to help the digestive tract protect us, and help protect us from invading organisms.

What Is Autoimmunity?

When immune cells mistakenly see your proteins, organs, body tissue hormones, neurotransmitters, and enzymes as harmful invaders, they attack them. People with autoimmunity have problems, and others can't see them. You can get image scans, lab tests, and they come back normal. Your symptoms are not advanced enough for medical diagnosis. If your doctor doesn't check for autoimmune markers, you will never be diagnosed. People out there aren't pushy enough to ask about their symptoms, and these symptoms become normal to them. They can suffer their whole life. I have been left, ignored, belittled, and made fun of by friends, family, and even doctors by complaining about my symptoms that seemingly have no explanation.

Doctors will prescribe an antidepressant to treat this mysterious disease. Luckily, today we have advanced testing that can detect whether you suffer from autoimmunity. Cyrex Labs is a clinical immunity laboratory specializing in immunology and autoimmunity. They will test twenty-four with one test things like gluten, allergies, Crohn's, and colitis. These tests may also find things you didn't know you had. It can alert you of brain disorders or joint problems that can paralyze you later in life and help you to be better prepared. You do have to ask your regular doctor to send you to this lab or order online. You can order a test at home through Everlywell.com.

Really Know What You're Eating

When I did try and get out and have a normal life with other people, it was great but hard to coordinate with them. It seemed like when my pain was at its worst; my friends were partying it up. When I was feeling great that day, they were nowhere to be found. My dating life was on and off again. If I ever went on a date, I was never available when they wanted to see me, and I was always running home. I didn't want to use the restroom there. I was never eating in front of them as my stomach would be in pain. Anything on a restaurant menu was not an option for my stomach.

I had a problem with restaurants when I questioned what kind of oil they use? They would give me the weirdest look. Like I was crazy. If they only knew that the oil was killing my gut, they might understand then. They're getting paid to serve us food that is good for you and tell us about the food. They are our lifeline with the very busy chefs. We are putting our allergies in their hands. If I asked about seafood allergies, they might have been ok with it. I have asked waiters if their avocados are fresh or come in a package? They'd say yes, it's fresh. I have gone through this multiple times, so I have no trust in them. The waiter thought fresh was using the packaged avocado mix, canola oil, and water, making it fresh every day. Premixed packages are high in Trans Fats. Companies use this fat to help preserve foods.

People have different visions of how to make fresh food, the same when I ask about oils being fresh. Some oils are wonderful for you but need to be used correctly. Store them in a dark, cool area not next to the stove, or leave them out in a hot kitchen when you store them for a long period. What happens when you heat it up? It then turns into a hydronated oil that is rancid for your stomach. Old oil is a harbor for free radicals. The oils oxidize over time and make you very sick. Instead, use small amounts of good oil, store in a dark, cool area, and discard them after six months. You need to use certain ingredients to make foods emulsify, bring out flavors, or not make them hurt you. Hydrogenated vegetable oils are manufactured by forcing hydrogen into the ingredients to increase their shelf life. As a result, the structure of the fat molecules is transformed in the opposite direction compared to natural fat molecules, turning into Trans-Fat. The fat will get lodged into your arteries, increase your risk of heart disease, inflammation, and raise your insulin level.

I would try this diet and did not understand the reason why this diet wasn't working for me. I had to stop myself and think about what food was real food or fake. Then I would eat it. Training yourself to do that was a challenge. When you're in a hurry and hungry, you have to be patient. It was easier for me because I knew it was going to hurt me. If you don't think before you eat you will suffer the consequences later.

CHAPTER 2

Eat to live, not live to eat— understanding what we put in our mouths is a part of us.

The only winners of the war on obesity are the corporations that sell diet food, diet pills, and other weight loss aids that are not working. When going on a diet, people usually start by lowering their fat intake or choosing low-fat foods. Doing this is not always the best choice. We get most of our nutrients from good fats. It helps us absorb nutrients better, gives us energy, and supports cell growth to heal our bodies. Not only are we taking out these good fats, but we are also adding in trans fats to preserve foods longer. Then we want to make them cheaper, so foods turn into fake food with no vitamins added to them. Think about where we get these nutritional vitamins and minerals from. They give us mixed messages about pills and vitamins and tell us it's the natural way to cure or get our daily vitamins.

Vitamins and minerals in supplements are synthetic forms of nutrients. Sometimes the usual forms found in multiple vitamin pills are identical to those found in foods. For a pill to absorb, it needs more vitamin e and the same with essential amino acids that can't absorb without certain vitamins. **For a pill to work, it must dissolve and disintegrate, and with all the stomach issues today, that doesn't happen very well.**

Here is a list of ways to tell you are getting good vitamins and minerals from supplements:

- Look for the USP symbol- US pharmacopeia/independent tested to make sure it will dissolve in your stomach well enough.
- Look for 100% whole food or daily value nutrients.
- Don't spend extra money on products that are marked high potency, stress formula, or a laboratory approved.
- Make sure that companies are not throwing in added vitamins you don't need and charge you for more.
- Always find out what you need and why it's helping you. Why waste money.

Food is always the best way to get nutrition unless you have an illness and need to add supplements with these foods. Foods contain other substances like vitamins and minerals for health. Fruit, vegetables, and whole grains contain vitamins, minerals, fiber, and phytochemicals which can help fight chronic disorders and cancers.

Now let's look at butter; butter was considered bad for you in the '80s. Now nutritionists are telling people to add butter to coffee. Choose grass-fed butter or Ghee, not margarine. This butter has good cholesterol, reduces fatty liver, keeps you fuller longer, and much more. Our bodies are brilliant. It knows which nutrients to use and cleanse the rest. The food industry is using science to make you crave food more. There's a report on CBC News from Kelly Crowe (Food cravings engineered by industry.)

Companies will use hydrogenated oils to improve shelf life and process them faster. When we use science to change our food, we can lose good nutrients from our food. If you use organic, unpasteurized butter, it will have many health benefits. Microorganisms are a natural way of sterilizing. These bugs are awesome for our bellies. The butter has vitamins A, E, and K2. It has Butyrate, which lowers Triglycerides, Insulin, and Conjugated Linoleic Acid, which is Omega-3 oil that controls inflammation, a necessity for chronic pain.

It has been shown to have anti-cancer properties as well as lowering body fat. People get very confused about this. They don't understand what pasteurized and unpasteurized mean. It makes a huge difference in your life. The heat kills these wonderful bugs (Enzymes) that eat all the food our bodies can't digest. Some of these bugs are fighting for you to survive.

The pro biotics that occurs in fermented foods like sauerkraut, kimchee, pickles, kefir are very beneficial to us. We can make soda fermented or make it out of almost anything. Back in the older times, Queen Cleopatra loved fermented foods. It was very big back then. Our generation lost that piece of great information along the way. Now pro biotics help rebalance your gut bugs by creating an environment where the good gut regains strength. Prebiotics are a food source for the microbes in your gut, which turns food into anti-inflammatory compounds.

Here are some foods that are prebiotic and or probiotic:

- **Dark chocolate** – 70 percent or higher.
- **Greek yogurt**
- **Organic green peas** – Helps the immune system to protect the mucosal barrier.
- **Sauerkraut** – reduce cholesterol levels.
- **Beer and wine** – beer decreases blood clot and wine has free radical fighting antioxidants.
- **Green olives** – makes stomach flatter, balance gut bugs, and bloating with IBS.
- **Natto fermented soybean** – healthiest food for woman and has the highest source of vitamin k2.
- **Sourdough bread** – yeast and friendly bacteria break down the gluten and sugar in the flour making it easier to digest.

Some products are heat-treated after fermentation, which kills most of the beneficial active cultures. Be sure to check the labels for the phrase "live active cultures."

We do know that our gut flora helps us properly digest our food, protects us from pathogens, helps us detoxify harmful compounds, produces vitamins, keeps our guts healthy, and balances our immune system.

The brain thrives when it`s nourished with essential fatty acids (omega 3s)

DHA is the most abundant fat in the brain. You can get a lot of this from cold wild fish. Not from farmed raised fish. Farm-raised fish live and eat in their own feces, and then you're eating that. Also, choose fish that are in the open, very cold oceans and have gills. Gills are like filters for the fish. It keeps the fish from being too acidic. The bottom feeders like Tilapia are the worst for you. Any fish without gills are not good for us to eat. They are bottom feeders. It makes your body so acidic and causes inflammation and possible cancer. That is why they are so cheap at the store.

To utilize these healthy fats, you must convert these sources to EPA and DHA. These are Omega-3 Fatty acids and are found in fatty layers of cold-water fish, plants, and nut oils. Omega-3 fatty acids are important fats you must get from your diet, as you can't produce them naturally. Omega-3 will lower inflammation in your body, and omega-6 could raise it. You will need vitamins and minerals to absorb these good fats and essential amino acids that our bodies are not able to absorb.

These vitamins can help with the process:

- Vitamin B12
- Thiamine
- Folate
- Vitamin B6
- Antioxidants
- Amino acids

You may think Vitamins are the least of your worries. I would love for us all to get these from whole foods, but you need supplements on top of whole foods when you're sick.

Science is now discovering that your gut will affect your brain health. Researchers have found a link between depression and gut inflammation.

Your body tells you when your brain is under attack by:

- Bloating
- Gas
- Pain
- Heartburn
- Diarrhea
- Constipation
- Food sensitivities

Your immune system is attacking you when this happens. You may think these are normal to have from all the commercials for heartburn and indigestion. When I get sharp pains in my stomach, that tells me to take omega-3 fish oil and enzymes. Within a few minutes, the pain should be better.

Another tummy soother that I use: Blend and heat coconut milk, Mint tea, Turmeric powder, and pepper on top. Drink every day when you have inflammation. That's my recipe for stomach issues, and it works like a charm.

Oils That Are Killing Us, And Why?

Hydrogenated vegetable oils are added to foods to keep costs low and long shelf life. Studies have shown that the trans-fat in these oils can increase inflammation in our bodies. Inflammation is normal for infection, but chronic inflammation is not, and these oils contribute to it. One of these oils I see a lot of is Canola oil. This oil is made from a canola plant that was crossbreed with rapeseed. This plant has high levels of erucic acid that is toxic to humans. Oils have certain heat temperatures or lifespan, or they become rancid and cause inflammation in our stomachs.

It's in everything like:

- Packaged snacks
- Baked goods
- Fried food
- Creamers both non-milk and milk
- Chips

These canola oils will get a wash of hexane solvent, sodium hydroxide, then bleached to lighten up the oil and steam injected to remove the bitter smell. Monounsaturated and polyunsaturated fats are healthy fats. These fats are liquid at room temperature and solid when chilled. If the butter is solid at room temperature, it is made with trans-fat to keep it solid.

Saturated and trans-fat are solid all the time. That's how you tell the difference. These are bad fats for you. When you grab two different bags of store-bought almonds and look at the nutrition facts, one bag will have only saturated and trans-fat. The other will have monounsaturated and polyunsaturated fats. Both are the same almond, but the ones with monounsaturated and polyunsaturated oils are better for you. The other is usually cheaper to buy. Just watch what you eat and **read the labels** on the back. We think we are eating organic chips but are hurting our stomachs from the canola oil in them.

NUTRITION FACTS

	% Daily Value*
Serving size	
Serving per Container	
Amount per serving	
Calories	
Total fat 20gr	10%
Saturated fat 15gr	8%
Cholesterol 8gr	4%
Sodium 2gr	1%
Total carbohydrate 7gr	3%
Dietary Fiber 5gr	4%
Sugar 10gr	5%
Protein 30gr	25%
Vitamin A 15%	Vitamin C 15%
Calcium 7%	Iron 5%

*Percent Daily values are based on 2.000 calories diet. Your daily values may be higher or lower depending on your calories needs.

Nutrition Facts

Serving		
10 Serving per Container		
Serving size		**2/3 cup (60g)**
Amount per serving		
Calories		**200**
		% Daily Value*
Total fat 10gr		
Saturated fat 5gr		
Cholesterol 15gr		
Sodium 10gr		15%
Total carbohydrate 5gr		8%
Dietary Fiber		20%
Total Sugars 12gr		5%
Protein 8gr		
Vitamin A 2mcg 12% • Calcium 120gr 5%		
Iron 8mg 30%		

*Percent Daily values are based on 2.000 calories diet. Your daily values may be higher or lower depending on your calories needs.

Here are some bad oils:

- **Soybean oil -** It has high levels of omega-6, which leads to chronic inflammation.
- **Corn oil -** It has omega-6 that outnumbers the omega-3 at a ratio of 49:1 needs to be 1:1.
- **Cottonseed oil -** It is made from GE cotton plants may cause your health to suffer.
- **Canola oil -** When consumed, it can introduce oxidized cholesterol and inflammation from Hexane into your body.

Here are good alternatives to utilize:

- **Olive oil -** It is used as unheated as a salad dressing.
- **Grass-fed butter -** It contains various nutrients and antioxidants that help your health.
- **Peanut oil -** It is consumed in small amounts unheated it`s high in omega-6.
- **Sesame oil -** In small amounts may help with symptoms of diabetes.
- **Coconut oil -** It is rich in healthy fats that can provide numerous benefits.

When people are on diets, they tend not to eat any fats at all, which is very bad for you. Healthy fats provide cell growth, give energy, lower blood sugar levels, and improve insulin control.

These good fats are essential fatty acids that your body needs for brain function and cell growth. Your body can't make essential fatty acids and must get them from your diet. These fats contain either omega-3, omega-6, or omega-9 fatty acids and are all important dietary fats. Omega-3 has EPA, DHA, and ALA. EPA's main function is to produce eicosanoids, which help reduce inflammation and depression. DHA's contribute to brain function and development. ALA's can convert to both and could benefit the heart, immune system, and nervous system. According to the National Institutes of Health, Omega-6 has Linoleic acid, and the body will convert to longer omega-6 fats like arachidonic acid, which are more pro-inflammatory.

Western diets consume too much omega-6, as companies use this fat to make food solid and last longer. Too much could cause a risk of inflammation and inflammatory disease. The omega-9 fatty acid is made in our bodies naturally, so they're non-essential.

We should try to consume these good fats naturally through foods, but people who have illnesses also need to add supplements. My favorite to consume is Nordic Naturals omega-3. Stores will sell omega-3, omega-6 and omega-9 supplements which you would only need if you get no fats at all.

What Does GMO Mean?

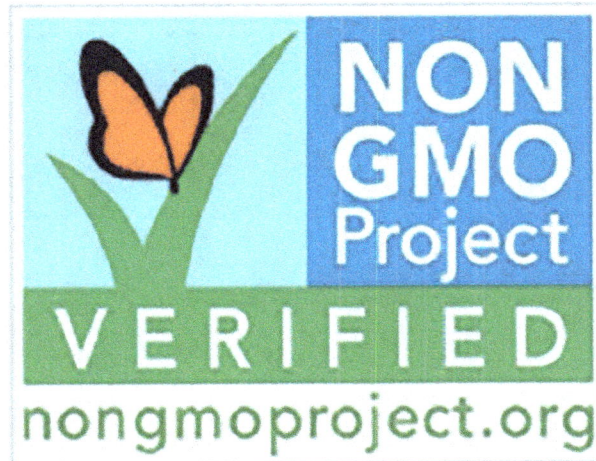

GMO, genetically modified organisms or plants that have been genetically altered in a laboratory through genetic engineering. These products do not exist naturally in nature. GMOs are designed to have more crop yield and are a strong defense against pests and drought issues. They have been linked to more health problems, including allergies, disturbances in the reproductive cycle, and certain cancers. A few examples are corn, soy, canola, safflower oil, and cottonseed oil.

GMO foods have been genetically altered by wiring in the DNA of pesticides and herbicides.

- Go on websites of grocery stores to see if they carry non-GMO products.
- Most frozen fruit/veggies are non-GMO
- Look for a seal of approval on the packages that say non-GMO and even organic.
- Read labels on the back of packages to see what is in them.
- Be careful they have made up new names for ingredients that may be the same.
- Some packages will say organic and not be organic.

These chemicals are judged on a case-by-case basis; the Canadian association of physicians for the environment called for removing GMO foods from the market pending long-term health studies.

Now testing of these varies by country, with some nations banning or restricting them and others permitting regulations. Countries like:

- United States
- Canada
- Lebanon
- Egypt

Only authorize GMO:

- European union
- Brazil
- China

In the US, the FDA determines that GMOs are generally recognized as safe and therefore do not require additional testing if the product is equivalent to the non-modified product. I have no idea why anyone would want these bad chemicals in their food. I do not want to be a Guinee pig with these chemicals anymore. We all need to ban together and stop contributing to these companies.

What Does Organic Mean?

Organic means came from living matter. The USDA states that the goal of organic foods and organic farming is to integrate cultural, biological, and mechanical practices. That fosters the cycling of resources, promotes ecological balance, and conserves biodiversity. Meaning the contents should have an ingredient list, and the contents should be 95% or more certified organic. Meaning it is free of synthetic additives like pesticides, chemical fertilizers, dyes and must not be processed using industrial solvents, irradiation, or genetic engineering.

Now here's where it gets tricky certified organic isn`t the only label you will see.

- 100% organic means all must meet the guidelines above.
- Made with organic means 70% or more remaining ingredients may not be foods with additives on a special list.

Now, these are such strict rules on organic. But when we genetically modify our foods now, that has a big impact on our bodies.

To learn more, please read:
Foodanimalconcernstrust.org

If you want to know what's in your food, then please consider proposition **37.** We lost it on November 6, 2012, ballot in California because we were told it was going to cost us more to buy groceries from the labeling, which is not true as they change their labels all the time and big companies like Coke, Pepsi, Monsanto, Kraft, Bayer, and many more paid a lot to make it not pass. If it had passed, we would have:

- Required labeling on raw or processed food offered for sale to consumers if the food is made from plants or animals with genetic material changed in specific ways.
- Prohibited labeling or advertising such food as "natural."
- Exempted from these requirement foods that are "certified organic; unintentionally produced with genetically engineered material; made from animals fed or injected with genetically engineered themselves; processed with or containing only small amounts of genetically engineered ingredients; administered for treatment of medical conditions; sold for immediate consumption such as in a restaurant; or alcoholic beverages."

James Wheaton, who filed the ballot language for the initiative, called it "The California Right to Know Genetically Engineered Food Act." We all did not fully understand what was happening. The result from the ballot that year was:

NO, on prop 37- 6,442,371 51.4%
YES, on prop 37- 6,088,714 48.6%

The supporters that want to keep us healthy and fought for prop 37 are:

- Organic consumer fund
- Mercola health resources
- Kent Whealy
- Nature`s path food
- Dr. Bronner`s magic soaps
- Mark Squire/Stillonger Trust
- Wehah Farms
- Ali Partovi
- Amy`s kitchen
- Great foods of America
- Alex Bogusky
- Clif Bar &co.
- Crop Cooperative
- Annie`s inc.
- Michael S. Funk
- Nutiva

The opponents were:

- Dr. Bob Goldberg National Academy of Sciences
- Jamie Johansson family farmer in California
- Betty Jo Toccoli, president of California small business association
- Jonnalee Henderson affiliated with the California farm bureau federation
- Dr. Henry I. Miller founding director of the office of Biotechnology of the food & drug Administration
- Tom Hudson, executive director of the California taxpayer protection Committee
- California Republican Party

As of November 3, 2012, about $45.6 million had been donated to not letting us know what was going into our food. Here are some of those companies that donated against prop 37 (no):

- E.I. Dupont De Nemours & co.
- Pepsico, Inc.
- Grocery Manufacturers Association
- Dow Agrisciences
- Bayer CropScience
- B.A. SF Plant Science
- Syngenta Co.
- Kraft Foods label
- Coca-Cola North America
- Nestle USA
- Conagra Foods
- General Mills
- Kellogg Company
- Smithfield foods
- Del Monte Foods
- Campbell`s soup
- Heinz foods
- Hershey Company
- The J.M. Smucker Company
- Bimbo Bakeries
- Ocean Spray Cranberries
- Mars food North America
- Council for Biotechnology Information
- Hormel foods
- Unilever
- Bumble Bee Foods
- Sara Lee
- Kraft Food Group
- Pinnacle foods
- Dean Foods Company
- Biotechnology Industry Organization
- Bunge North America
- McCormick & co.
- Wm. Wrigley Jr. Company
- Abbott Nutrition
- Cargill Inc.
- Rich Products Corp.
- Flowers Foods
- Dole Packaged Foods
- Knouse Foods Cooperative

Other companies that donated but less than $150,00 were:

- Sunny Delight Beverages
- McCain foods
- Tree Top
- Idahoan Foods
- Richelieu Foods
- Land O Lakes
- Hillshire Brands
- Morton Salt
- Clorox
- Goya de Puerto Rico
- Sargento
- Godiva Chocolatier

We all need a better understanding of what we are voting for. People will listen to politics and money. We then will deal with the consequences later.

When you are buying from these companies, you are supporting them. Please support the smaller companies that are fighting for our health.

Plants Can Hurt Us

Lectins are in plants and meat. When the animal eats the plants and then we eat them, we are consuming these lectins. There are thousands of different kinds of Lectins. Among one Lectin, we call it gluten. A lot of people are allergic to gluten. Plants are protecting themselves and their offspring from hungry insects by producing toxins, including Lectins, in the plants' seeds and other parts. These toxins can kill or immobilize an insect can also silently destroy your health.

It's a good idea to chat with your doctor about starting an elimination diet that removes lectins. You should always listen to your body and see if a lectin-free diet could be right for you. To reduce lectins in your favorite foods, you can soak them overnight; it will help them reduce their plant lectins. You can use a pressure cooker or peel the skins and deseed them. Fermentation also allows good bacteria to get in there and break down some of the plant's defenses. Studying up the difference between high and low lectin foods will help you make the best choice. Learn what foods have lectins and how to stay away from them.

A plant may be good for one person but may hurt another person. Our stomachs are not all on the same strength levels as other stronger stomachs. You can slowly add it into your diet and train your cells to handle it and not hurt you, as we all need to learn to adapt to a new environment to be able to survive. This could be some of the reasons why our stomachs are hurting. Make sure to write down what is hurting you and what is good for you on your food log. To learn more about lectins, try reading The Plant Paradox by Steven R. Gundry, MD.

Intermitting Fasting

Our guts need to rest at certain times. Intestines are constantly pushing things through our bodies. It also produces various substances that carry messages to other body parts, fights germs, and regulate the body's water balance. During intermittent fasting, the gut microbiome gets a good rest from breaking down food to keep our system running properly.

Fasting and diet changes can alter the composition and population of microbes in the gut. Even specific food groups cause noticeable changes. Research supports the connection between our circadian rhythms and our gut microbiomes which also affect our sleep cycle. Intermittent fasting will help our body composition, sleep cycles, blood glucose, longevity, and even inflammation. Intermittent fasting is a pattern of eating, and it will reduce insulin hormone by 20 to 30 percent, making it easier to control weight loss and increase your metabolism. Every time you eat, even healthy food will spike your insulin levels.

Ideally, you want to start out by fasting for 16 hours and eating within an 8-hour window. Then gradually move to 20 hours and within a 4-hour window. An easier way to look at it is to go to bed at 9, sleep for 16 hours and wake up without eating. Don't eat until 12 pm. Eat at 12 pm and then eat again at 4 pm then start the fast again. Remember to eat a good monounsaturated fat with your meal. It will help your cell membranes to repair and keep you less hungry. Your body will realize it's going into starvation, and your body will adjust itself if you have no food for stretches of time. Your body breaks down food into glucose. Glucose provides energy to the body to help it survive. After 8 to 12 hours, your glucose storage is depleted. Your body will begin to convert glycogen from your liver and muscles into glucose. After this is depleted, your body will begin to use amino acids to provide energy, then metabolism shifts to preserve lean body tissue, and to prevent muscle loss, the body begins to rely on fat stores to create ketones for energy, a process known as ketosis. You will experience weight loss during this time. You can learn more about fasting from Dr. Eric Berg. He has some great youtube video tutorials on how to fast correctly. A good way to control what you eat is by growing your organic farm.

You can save money by doing your own garden and using these techniques for pesticides.

- Tomatoes, garlic, chives, mint, basil, and cilantro will steer pests away just from their smell.
- Ladybugs and many other good bugs eat the other bus.
- Cedar, salts, pine needles, and even human hair bugs hate too.
- Chickens eat mosquitos and bugs.
- Chili peppers, cat litter, and sour tasting plants in front of the regular plants will keep them away naturally.
- You can wash your produce with a mixture of vinegar, lemon, and baking soda to clean them.
- Lemon, vinegar, honey, and salts help preserve the food.
- You can disinfect with vinegar, ultra-lights, and heat.
- Keep your produce in the dark area and put it in an air-tight container.

If you have land, that is great, but there are still ways to grow Veggies without land if you don't. Aeroponics is the process of growing plants in the air or mist environment without the use of soil. You can buy these online; they do get pricey but work very well. You can even grow a garden in an apartment with containers and soda bottles.

I would recycle a soda bottle and hang from above and let the tomato grow downwards, and I would save my leftover stumps from veggies and put them in a jar with water and grow new roots. The more you learn, the better the garden gets.

Let's face it, your weekly run to the store is the next foundation for your good health. It's amazing news that the supermarket industry is on a health kick. Go on their website and look for the deals. Sprout, Wholefoods, Baron's, Jimbo's, Windmill, Trader Joe's, Farmers Markets, and many others are here to help in the journey to a healthy body.

CHAPTER 3

Essentials of Life

The first place you want to start is to find out if you have digestive issues or an allergy reaction. Eat something and then wait for 30 minutes and see if you are having allergies or digestive issues. Here are a few signs:

- Breathing hard /can`t catch your breath
- Coughing, itching any part of the body
- Rashes / red patches on the skin
- Allergies

The body is constantly exposed to infections, but diseases only occur when an organism overwhelms the immune system's attempts to overcome it.

These organisms can enter through your skin by a cut or injury through the mucous membranes of the eyes, nose, ears, digestive tract, and lungs. They may spread in the bloodstream, along nerves, or by invading body tissues. Most of these pathogens are living organisms, and when they enter the body, the immune system gives a response to fight them off. These responses will give symptoms of illness, such as fever, inflammation, and increased production of mucous. The severity of the disorder depends on the strength and numbers of the invading organisms and the host's immune response. Some infections last only a short time before either defeat by the host's defenses or the host's death. Others become **CHRONIC.**

- Nonstop digesting for long times
- Pain like a sharp object feeling going down the stomach.
- Diarrhea
- Food not digesting or going down
- Nausea
- Allergy

The digestion process produces simple nutrients that provide the raw materials for metabolism. These collected chemical reactions working together will make the cells alive.

You can still do some tests with your doctor, or you can order the test through the mail at EverlyWell.com and Biodome.com. These tests will tell you what`s inside of you and if it`s hurting you.

You can also do:

1. Get a food diary for the month.
2. Get diagnostic labs done.
3. Hair mineral and skin analysis

Lab test you should examine:

What to test	What it is testing
1. Nutritional status	pathogens, low amino acid,
2. Digestive function	pathogens, stress, nutritional deficiency
3. Food/environment allergy	learning, behavior problems, rash, acne
4. Gastrointestinal pathogens	Bacteria, yeast, candida, acne
5. Amino acid balance	nutritional deficiency, allergy, pathogens
6. Energy metabolism	low amino acid, low protein, pathogens, stress
7. Hormone balance	stress, bacteria, enzymes

You will need to ask your doctor to test for these problems. If the doctor doesn't approve of it, then your insurance won't pay for it. You would need to pay for it online. If I had done this first, I would have fixed most of my pain and paid less to my insurance company.

I see why they possibly might be a little quiet about it. Not all doctors are like this, there are a lot trying to help us. Doctors don`t want to bombard you with tests either unless you ask. Some doctors are trying to get knowledge on this health kick. Not only did they go to school for a long time, but the doctors are also going outside of their training to educate themselves on stuff that is not in their area of work to help us. That would be for a Bacteriologist or a Toxicologist. We thank you for that.

Here is some test that will help you in finding what is wrong with you. You may have to use a holistic doctor or order online.

Hair mineral skin analysis test is the most accurate way to analyze exposure to heavy metals, low absorption of minerals. The hair analysis is effective compared to a blood test because your body carefully regulates the mineral levels free-floating in the bloodstream, meaning the blood test results generally do not show the true body level. The rest of the mineral gets stored in organs and tissues, such as the hair. You can order this test to be sent to you **Evenbetterhealth.com will mail you the test.**

Saliva testing can accurately measure levels of hormones such as DHEA, progesterone, testosterone, and estrogen. Most blood tests don't come close enough to this test on checking hormones. Saliva hormone testing reflects how your tissues absorb and respond to hormones delivered topically through the skin in creams, gels, or patches.
Some doctors will talk you into doing a blood and urine test for this. But blood and urine testing underestimate hormones delivered topically. Ask for the saliva test.

Food sensitivity test not to be confused with the allergy test. 96 common foods found in modern western diet, including gluten, dairy, wheat, and yeast. Many of us don't understand what this is. If you're wheezing after a meal, then you are having an attack.

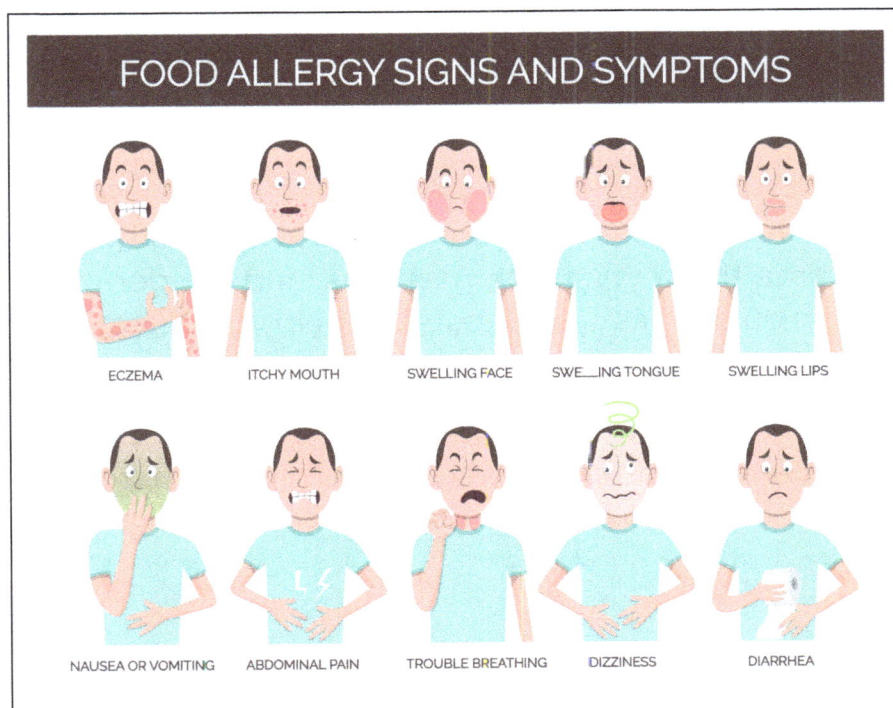

FOOD ALLERGY SIGNS AND SYMPTOMS

ECZEMA ITCHY MOUTH SWELLING FACE SWE__ING TONGUE SWELLING LIPS

NAUSEA OR VOMITING ABDOMINAL PAIN TROUBLE BREATHING DIZZINESS DIARRHEA

Iridology test. Patterns, color, and other characteristics of the iris can be examined to determine information about a patient's systemic health. Practitioners match their observations to iris charts. They can tell your mom's DNA side of the family and dad's side too. Then also tell you what is causing the damage now. Iridology seeks out potential and developing diseases before they become a symptom. An Iridologist is an individual that has been trained in all seven Iridology, and Sclerology-these time honored health evaluation methods make up what is called Iridology.

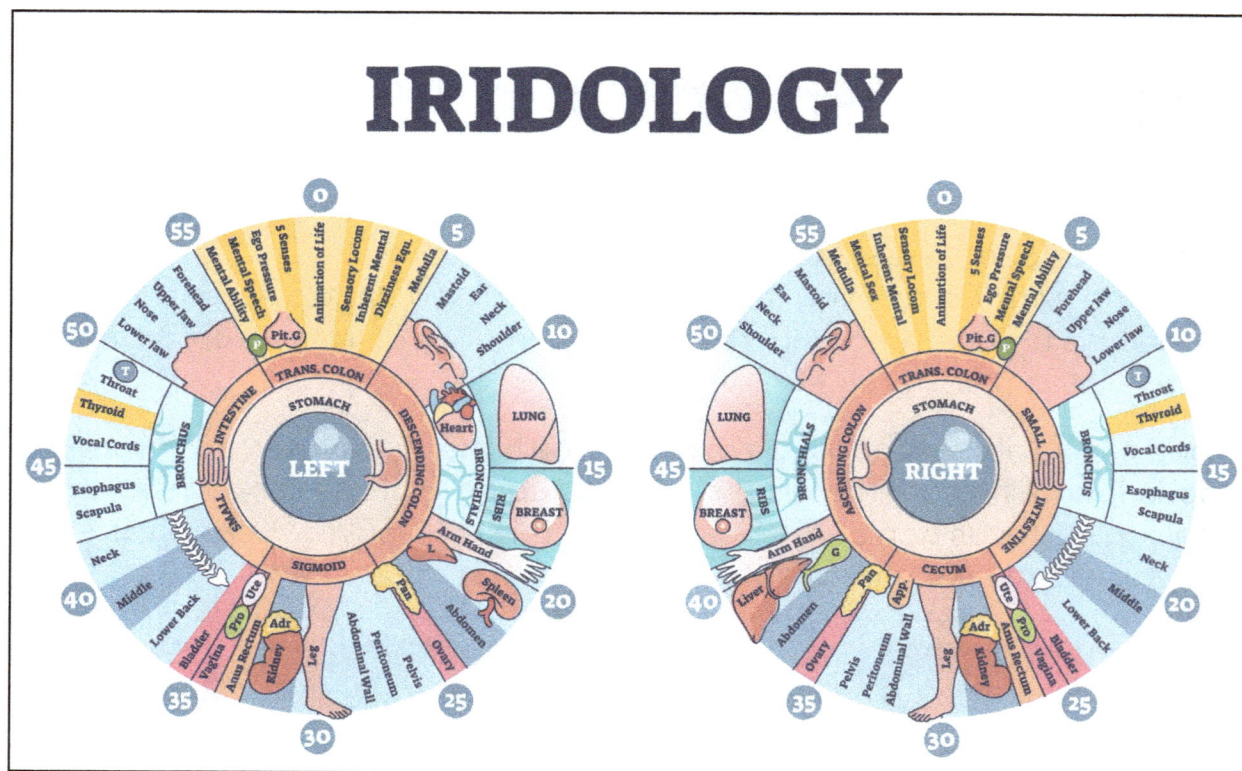

Mostly everyone has a lead, mold, aluminum, and many other things in their system. Over time these will block passages, and we don`t get our daily nutrients to heal our bodies. These tests will help you detect any problems.

The Acidic Test - will tell you if the food you are eating is too acidic for you. When you are too acidic, your body won't heal and could cause you cancer. It tests the level and the amount of acid in the stomach. Your body needs to be in an alkaline state to heal. If you are acidic, then change your diet to the acidic diet.

pH scale

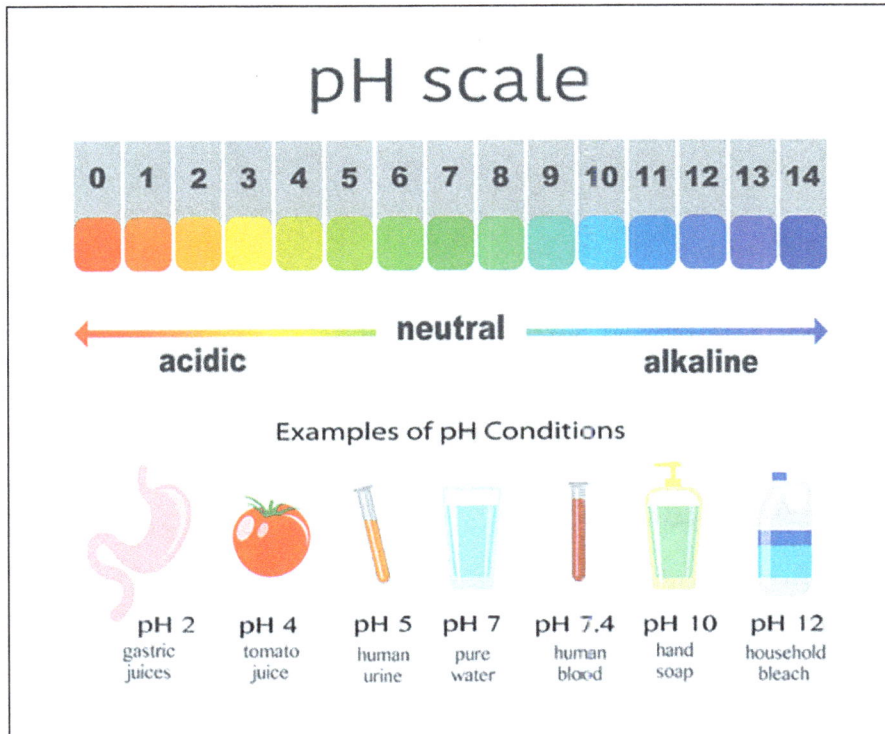

| 0 | 1 | 2 | 3 | 4 | 5 | 6 | 7 | 8 | 9 | 10 | 11 | 12 | 13 | 14 |

neutral

acidic — alkaline

Examples of pH Conditions

pH 2	pH 4	pH 5	pH 7	pH 7.4	pH 10	pH 12
gastric juices	tomato juice	human urine	pure water	human blood	hand soap	household bleach

What Are Minerals, And Why Do We Need Them?

Minerals are remnants of rocks, sand, and decomposed plants, animals, and humans. They play a role in the maintenance of your body's metabolic function and growth. Minerals are actual elements in their simple, inorganic form.

Minerals Consist Of:

- Phosphorus
- Iodine
- Magnesium
- Zinc
- Copper
- Selenium
- Chloride
- Potassium

What Are Amino Acids?

They play central roles both as building blocks of proteins and as intermediates in metabolism. The 20 amino acids that are found within proteins convey a variety of chemical versatility.

The ten amino acids that we can produce are:

- Alanine
- Glutamic acid
- Glutamine
- Glycine
- Proline
- Asparagine
- Aspartic acid
- Cysteine
- Serine
- Tyrosine

What Are Essential Nutrients?

Humans can produce 10 of the 20 amino acids. The others must be supplied from the food. Failure to obtain enough of even one of the ten essential amino acids will degrade the body's proteins, muscles, and so forth to obtain the one needed amino acid.

- Arginine
- Histidine
- Isoleucine
- Leucine
- Lysine
- Methionine
- Phenylalanine
- Threonine
- Tryptophan
- Valine

These amino acids are required in the diet. Plants, of course, must be able to make all the amino acids. People do not have all the enzymes required for the biosynthesis of all the amino acids.

Protein

Protein is found all through the body- in muscle, bone, skin, hair, and every other body part or tissue. It makes up the enzymes that help many chemical reactions and the hemoglobin that carries the oxygen in your body. At least 10,000 different proteins make you what you are and keep you that way. You need 8 grams of protein for every 20 pounds of body weight. Animal protein sources will deliver all the amino acids we need; other proteins, such as fruits, veggies, grains, nuts, and seeds, lack one or more essential amino acids. There is evidence that high-protein food choices play a role in health. Eating healthy protein sources like fish, chicken, beans, or nuts in place of red meat can lower the risk of several diseases and premature death.

Nucleic Acid

It will store genetic information that you got from your parents. If you have children, your genes will be recombined with your partner`s genetic information to show genetic information that will be stored in the nucleus of every cell in your child`s body. If you don`t want to pass down diseases to your child, you should consider iridology and amino acids to help fix that.

What Are Vitamins?

They are chemical compounds found in different food sources that are essential for the body to function. We have 13 vitamins that our bodies can`t produce, so we need food and supplements to provide them. They regulate your blood, help you convert fat and carbs into energy, protect cells from damage, and assist in the formation of new cells, bones, and tissue.

The vitamins are:

- Vitamin A
- Vitamin C
- Vitamin D
- Vitamin E
- Vitamin K
- Vitamin B1
- Vitamin B2
- Vitamin B6
- Vitamin B12
- Niacin
- Folate
- Biotin
- Pantothenic Acid

We divide these into two groups known as fat-soluble vitamins and water-soluble vitamins.

- **Fat-soluble** Vitamin A, D, E, and K. These are absorbed through the lymphatic system. Then drained into the bloodstream to be stored in the liver and fatty tissue. Needed in small doses.
- **Water-soluble** Vitamin B and C. These are easily dissolved and can be excreted in the urine. Needed in small, frequent doses.

These vitamins listed above have an important job in the body.

A vitamin deficiency occurs when you do not get enough of a certain vitamin. The difference between these two groups is how each vitamin acts within the body. Fat-soluble vitamins dissolve in fats to absorb the nutrients better. A low-fat diet can cause a deficiency. Water-soluble vitamins are needed for their functions, health benefits, and dietary sources.

What Are Electrolytes?

Both vitamins are important; however, cutting out good fats and having illnesses interfere with the absorption of vitamins. A few disorders that interfere are autoimmune disease, diarrhea, blockage of bile ducts, weight loss, bariatric surgery, liver disorder, alcoholism, and drugs. Water-soluble minerals that carry electrically charged potassium and chloride. Which are carried by fluids that help enable proper cellular and organ functions. You can lose them through sweating, and they affect the amount of water in your body and muscle functions. *Potassium* keeps your nutrients moving in and waste flowing out of your cells. *Chloride* helps with maintaining your body's proper balance of body fluids and is an essential part of your digestive juices.

Now looking at plants, we need the same nutrients as plants. The only difference is that plants can make their own nutrients and food. We can't. They use photosynthesis- plants and organisms convert light into energy that can later be released to fuel them.

The body can heal itself, but sometimes it needs help. Our bodies have an amazing capacity to heal and are the most important bodily functions, right next to regulating blood pressure and digesting our food. The best approach is to restore this natural mechanism. All human life originally begins as one single cell. Every second that we're alive, the cells in our bodies work to bring us back to our natural health. When we use medicine to heal us, we are weakening our body's natural ability to heal. Each cell is always working to heal and adjust its process, restoring itself according to the original DNA code it was created with to maintain balance within the body.

You can have a whole new body every 7 to 10 years. Every cell in your body is replaced by a new cell. When a human dies, it may take hours or a day before all the cells in the body die (this is what the forensic investigators go by when determining the time and death.) Our bodies are so amazing we just need to find the clues.

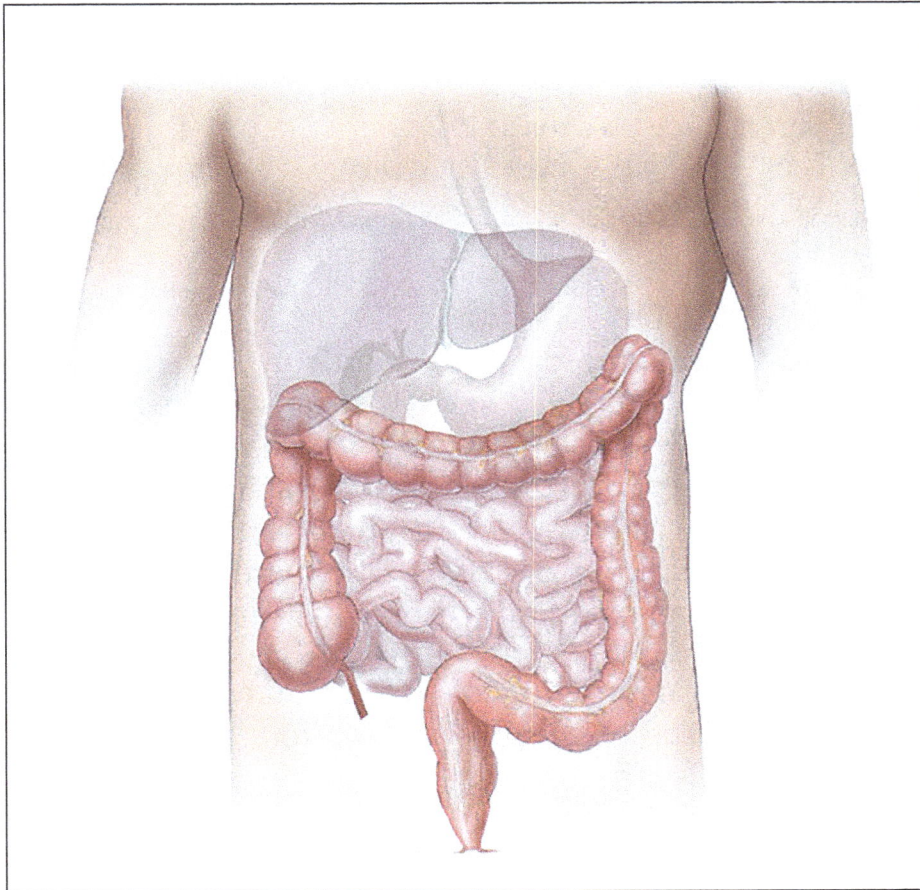

Suck out that poop!

When our bodies are healthy, it produces toxins. Our bodies need to eliminate these toxins. Even if you don't put toxins in your body, it will create waste material and toxins. When toxins are accumulated, they cause the immune system to suppress, and the body becomes acidic. The acidic body lets illness and disease grow. Get rid of this, and your body will be alkaline and heal. Our bodies get messed up from all this pollution, chemicals, pesticides that kill our good bugs, and so much more.

The reason we get sick is:

- Your body is out of balance.
- Your immune system is not functioning properly.
- Toxins are getting into your body.
- Not functioning very well.

Cleanse this stuff out, and your body will run again properly.

We can eliminate through:

- **Nose -** It eliminates using lungs.
- **Mouth -** It eliminates using lung.
- **Urinary Tract -** It eliminates through kidneys and liver.
- **Colon -** It eliminates through the liver, stomach, and small intestines.
- **Skin -** It eliminates through perspiration.

Poop, Yes, I said it.

The colon's most important role is to act as a magnet and push the waste out. It can then reabsorb water and salts through sodium and chloride, just like an electric charge. This will help the body maintain its normal water content, avoid dehydration, and transform the watery waste into solid feces that are easier to move and dispose of. (Bentonite clay added to your fiber drink is a good way or eating a banana with a glass of water.) These items both have potassium and chloride in them.

When your bowel movements come too much or not enough, it can make you uncomfortable, bloated, or even interfere with your body`s ability to absorb enough nutrients.

3 Types of Movement:

1. *Segmentation* – Both nerves and muscles work together to create a rhythm. This rhythm helps absorb nutrients. Like, when a stone hits the water, it creates a wave or motion that pushes things along. But when a second one is dropped in, movement changes to up and down, appearing to stay in the same place. Diarrhea segmentation activity is too low, while constipation is too high.

2. *Peristalsis* - When you eat your meal, the food moves through your intestines by peristalsis. During this movement, your muscles contract and relax, allowing your food and liquids to be mixed and

move through your digestive tract. Think of the waves of the ocean. This helps the absorption of water and electrolytes.

3. *Mass movement* – A type of motility not seen elsewhere in the digestive tube. Very intense and prolonged peristaltic contraction, which strips an area of the large intestine clear of contents. Several times a day, mass movement push feces into the rectum, which is usually empty.

It takes 12 to 36 hours for this waste to go from the small intestine to the rectum. These movements are produced by the contractions of a layer of circular muscle. The strength of the colon contractions will be greater when you eat more fiber or veggies.

We have many conditions that make this not work properly. Spastic colon (IBS) is the spontaneous contractions or loss of muscle movement in the small and large intestines. Breathing in and exhaling a few times will help you relax the colon and release without any stress to the body. Lactose intolerance is when you cannot digest the main sugar found in milk and other dairy products. This is caused by lactase deficiency, the enzyme responsible for metabolizing lactose in the small intestines. People cannot produce lactase enzymes because of illness or injury in the small intestine, including surgery or infections. A hydrogen breath test is an inexpensive, easy way of determining if you are lactose intolerant. Constipation is when your poop is dry and gets stuck. Your muscles get hurt from sickness or disease and don`t work properly. Or you are not drinking enough water and fiber. We should try and drink at least one or more bottles of water a day.

We are all usually deficient in magnesium. It may be one of the most necessary supplements there is. It`s involved in 300 Biochemical functions in the body, such as regulating the heartbeat rhythms. It`s extremely important for your metabolism, enzyme function and for balancing Nitric Oxide in the body. It`s believed that magnesium in Citrate, Chelate, and Chloride forms is absorbed better than Magnesium sulfate.

Citrate: Laxative effect when taken in high doses but safe for improving digestion and preventing constipation.
Chelate: It is found in foods naturally. This type is bound to multiple amino acids(proteins) and used to restore magnesium levels.
Chloride oil: It helps with the absorption of magnesium from their food. Athletes will use to increase energy, endurance, dull muscle pain, and heal wounds.

To learn more, check out the website *Listen to Your Gut* by *Jini Patel*. She is amazing and was one of the first ones to discover our gut issues.

Face Mapping:

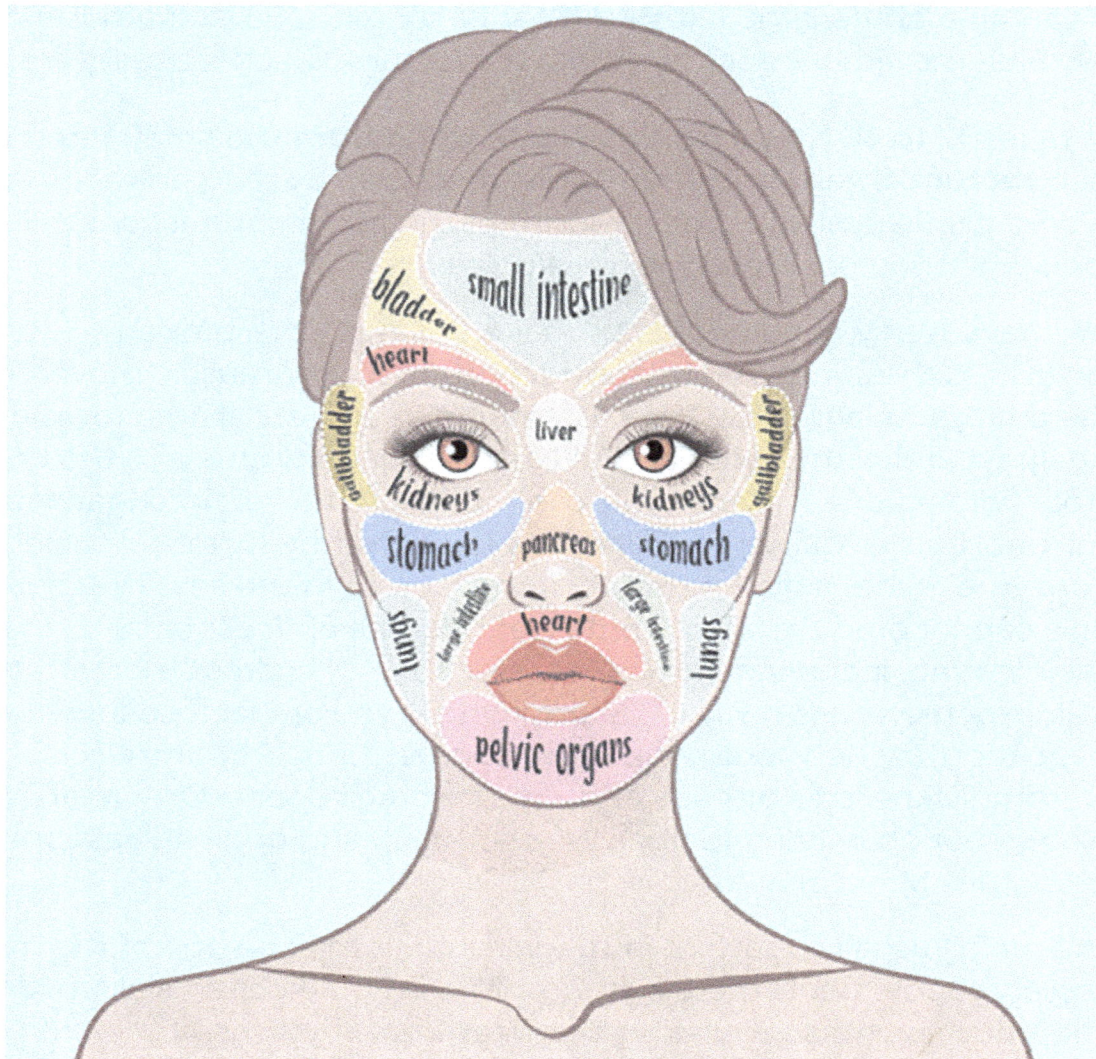

Google maps are working on using their services to map the cells in our bodies to help us heal. It's amazing what technology is doing now to help us heal. They are now using the technology on hip tissue to understand osteoarthritis and chronic joint pain better, but researchers hope to do the same with other tissues soon. For now, we use our bodies' different signs to help us. For instance, when we get dry skin, brittle nails, different colors of the skin, dry hair, and so on.

Some dermatologists can diagnose a problem by simply looking at your face and using a face mapping technique. It's a popular method in ancient Chinese medicine that focuses on the different areas of your face. Judging by the location of the acne or flare-up, doctors can determine its underlying cause. This is called Mien Shiang, which translates to face reading. It is a 3,000-year-old practice. The location of these blemishes on the face supposedly represents the organ that's affected.

Here are a few face mapping breakdowns.

Forehead:

When acne is present here, it could be caused by many issues, including digestive problems, small intestine problems, liver problems, high levels of stress, irregular sleep patterns, poor diets, and reactions to hair products. To combat forehead acne, get at least 7 hours of sleep, drink plenty of water to flush out toxins.

Temples/eyebrows/between brows:

Acne in this area can be due to poor circulation, gallbladder problems, or diets too high in fats, processed foods, or alcohol. Again, water intake is essential, as is watching one's diet and hygiene practices.

Nose:

Acne on the nose can be due to poor diet, constipation, bloating, gastrointestinal imbalance, indigestion, or poor blood circulation. Vitamin B, less seasoned foods, and massaging the nose area can help.

Mouth/Lip Area:

Acne here can be caused by constipation, spicy foods, and a reaction to a certain toothpaste. An increased intake of fiber, fruits, and veggies can help your skin.

Chin:

Hormonal problems can cause acne here, gynecological issues, kidney imbalance, touching skin, or toothpaste. Again, rest and water intake help plenty. You can take omega-3s to keep hormones in balance.

Another map is the Bristol stool chart helps with mapping your stomach issues. It is a diagnostic tool designed to classify the form of human feces into categories. It evaluates the effectiveness of treatments for various diseases of the bowel.

Here is an illustration to better help you understand:

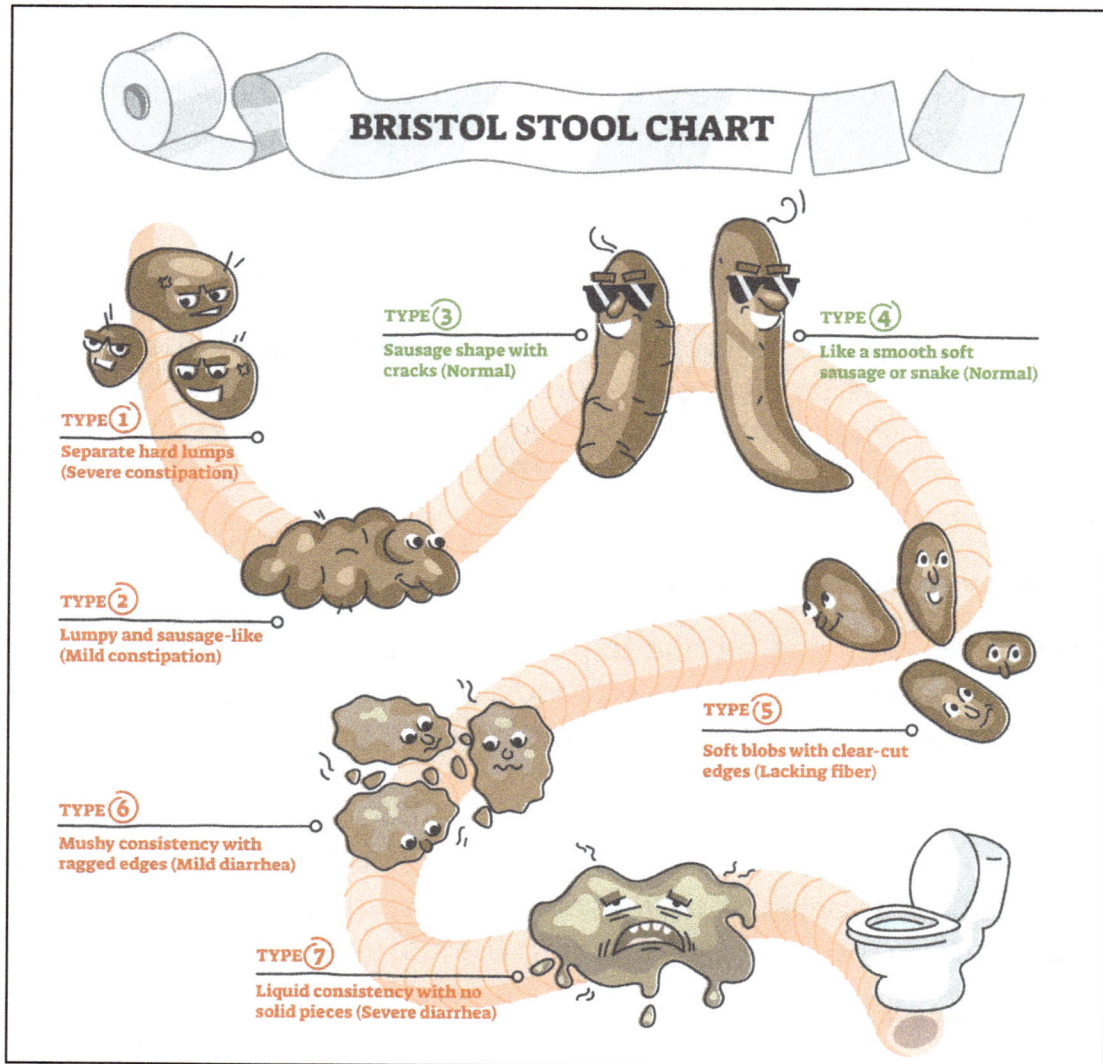

It was developed by Ken Heaton, MD, at the Bristol Royal infirmary as a clinical assessment tool in 1997 and is used widely as a tool to evaluate the effectiveness of treatments for various diseases. The Bristol scale is being used today at the Kaiser Permanente medical care program in San Diego, California. This tool helps doctors measure the time it takes for food to pass through your body and leave waste. The shape and form of your poop may also point your doctor towards a diagnosis of some digestive problems. Being in the middle of the chart is where you want to be. Different colors also help you to determine diseases too. It starts with normal, well-hydrated colors. But as you move down the list, dehydration becomes more severe. It can also tell you how acidic you are or how alkaline you are. Then you can change your diet to better your body.

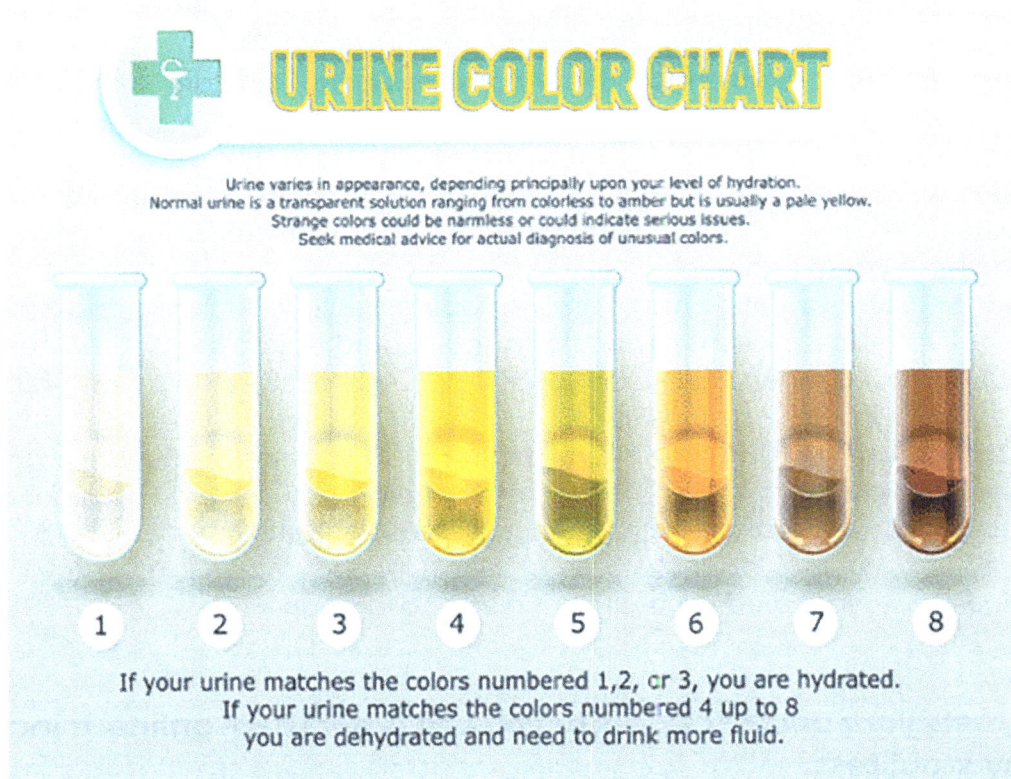

URINE COLOR CHART

Urine varies in appearance, depending principally upon your level of hydration.
Normal urine is a transparent solution ranging from colorless to amber but is usually a pale yellow.
Strange colors could be harmless or could indicate serious issues.
Seek medical advice for actual diagnosis of unusual colors.

1 2 3 4 5 6 7 8

If your urine matches the colors numbered 1,2, or 3, you are hydrated.
If your urine matches the colors numbered 4 up to 8
you are dehydrated and need to drink more fluid.

Urine has been a useful tool for diagnosing since the earliest days of medicine. When you're healthy and hydrated, your urine should be between clear and the color of light straw or honey. Change to severe dehydration can turn urine the color of amber. But urine can turn colors far beyond what's normal, including red, blue, green, dark brown, and cloudy white. Knowing your pee color will help and letting your doctor know when it changes color. I do feel our bodies work in amazing ways, and if you understand your body, it can help you heal it. Knowing what's in our bellies also will help with issues. Our bodies can get bacteria, parasites, and inflammation just from the food we eat.

Here are a few bacteria's you should test for before doing any drastic surgeries:

- **Giardia** - a parasite that infects the small intestine(ileum), causes inflammation, won't let you absorb proper nutrients. Patients suffer from chronic fatigue, depression, upper back, neck, and shoulder pain.
- **Helicobacter Pylori** - Infection in your stomach caused by gastritis and peptic ulcers. If you get tested for parasites, include a culture and sensitivity test for bacterial pathogens and H.pylori. Bacteria feed on undigested dietary protein, robbing your amino acids. Harmful bacteria develop when you have taken antibiotics.
- **Gut Microbiota** - Microorganisms including bacteria, archaea, and fungi that live in the digestive tracts of humans and animals (good bacteria that our bodies need). Specific probiotics are needed to help reestablish healthy bacteria in the intestines.
- **Clostridium Difficile** - Inflammation of the colon caused by the bacteria can be transmitted from person to person by spores. It usually develops after surgery and causes food and sugar to move through the stomach into your bowel too quickly. The body won`t break down or digest, preventing efficient digestion and absorption.

These tests your doctor can do, or you can order them online. It includes a 4-day stool test.

You would test for:

- Pathological yeast
- Parasites
- Parasite ova
- Bacteria
- Clostridium difficile
- E. Histolitica
- Giardia
- Colitis toxins A and B
- H. Pylori

Cleansing is a good way to reset your ecosystem.

Detox or cleanse is when you eliminate solid foods, so your digestive system is given a break, allowing it to heal and better absorb nutrients. You can push these toxins out faster by drinking water with lemon or water with maple syrup and cayenne pepper, and it will help aid the process. Your liver then will filter toxins and unwanted byproducts from your blood and will deliver nutrients to the body.

Detoxification means cleansing the blood. This is done by removing impurities from the blood and the liver, where the toxins are processed for elimination. The body eliminates toxins through the kidneys, intestines, lungs, lymphatic system, and skin. When these systems are compromised, impurities aren`t properly filtered, and the body is adversely affected.

A detox program can help the body's natural cleansing process by:

- Resting the organs through fasting.
- Stimulating the liver to drive toxins from the body.
- Promoting elimination through the intestines, kidneys, and skin.
- Improving circulation through the blood.
- Refueling the body with healthy nutrients.

Cleanses that need to be done at least once every five years.

- Liver/ Gallbladder cleanse
- Kidney cleanse
- Colon cleanse

Colonics is a procedure where you get three to fifteen pounds of undigested fecal matter out of your body that got stuck in your colon. This matter is highly toxic, suppressing your immune system, causing gas, bloating, constipation, and not absorbing your nutrients.

Getting this done will help with your anxiety, depression, stress, fatigue, constipation, hair, skin, and nails.

Now that you're all cleaned out start by:

- Adding in your minerals and vitamins.
- Eat organic veggies and fruit.
- Eat organic grass-fed meats.
- No cheese or milk products until you have a good amount of enzymes.
- Listen to meditation at night to sleep better and fix anxiety.
- No bread or sugar.

Digesting food takes anywhere from 24 to 72 hours, depending on the type of food and the presence of digestive issues.

Digestion begins when food enters the mouth, the food is mixed with stomach acid. Once in the small intestine, the food remnants are exposed to digestive juices, bile, and enzymes from the pancreas and liver. The food will move through the stomach and small intestines within 6 to 8 hours. Your intestines are long and winding so that your food can digest in a certain time. It helps the body to absorb better. When we have surgery and cut out parts of our intestines, our body will not absorb these nutrients correctly.

CHAPTER 4

Quick tips for fast healing
from probiotics and yeast

Babies receive beneficial bacteria from their mothers during vaginal birth and breast milk. We have about 7 pounds of bacteria in us. We are still discovering new probiotics today, but we believe we have over 100 trillion bacteria living in us. Each culture has different probiotics that help one person or could hurt another person.

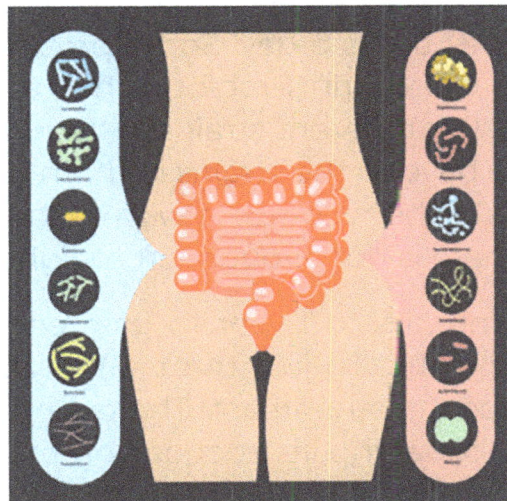

These are good bacteria that are protecting us. These bugs can repel harmful microbes and bacteria by repopulating the gut with healthy organisms. We have different strains of bugs that can heal certain chronic pains. The two most popular strains are Lactobacillus and Bifidobacterium. Probiotics will fight each other and need to be separated when taken but are great with prebiotics.

We have different species that can help us to be smarter, prettier, calmer, as they can change who we are. We have prebiotics, probiotics, and enzymes, and each one plays a different role in our bodies. Enzymes are molecules that assist in the breakdown of foods, and probiotics are living microorganisms that live in our gut and positively affect our body and physiological process. Prebiotics are high-fiber foods that act as food for human microflora.

What Are Probiotics?

The human GI tract naturally contains trillions of bacteria. These bacteria have many roles in our body, and having the correct balance of good bacteria is essential for keeping us healthy. Many problems can impact the type and number of bacteria in the gi tract by getting older, antibiotic use, IBs, and gastroenteritis. Probiotics are one way to help balance your GI tract. They are good bacteria found in certain foods and supplements, which have beneficial effects on our health.

How To Use Probiotics:

Start by ¼ tsp. for a month. If your stomach can handle it, then work your way up to three (3) times a day. You want to be taking three single, separate strains three (3) times a day. Some probiotics will be sold with different bugs in one pill. Natrin Probiotics has a patent on their pills. They have one pill that has different strains in them and is released when needed. Other pills will have all the strains in them and be released at the same time. This will make them compete with each other, and by the time they get to your gut, there is not enough left to fight.

Do this for six (6) months to 1 year to gain enough bugs to have a good colony. I noticed results in just three (3) days. No sugar while you do this. Sugar only helps the other team. There is no proper way of taking probiotics, but please follow the instructions on the bottle. I used Natrin probiotics, and they have strains that have patents on them that work amazingly. You can order them from www. natrin.com.

These bugs saved me from pain and will save you. If you are still in disbelief of this, then read Good Germs, Bad Germs by Jessica /Snyder Sachs. It explains in detail all about probiotics and is one of my favorite ones to read.

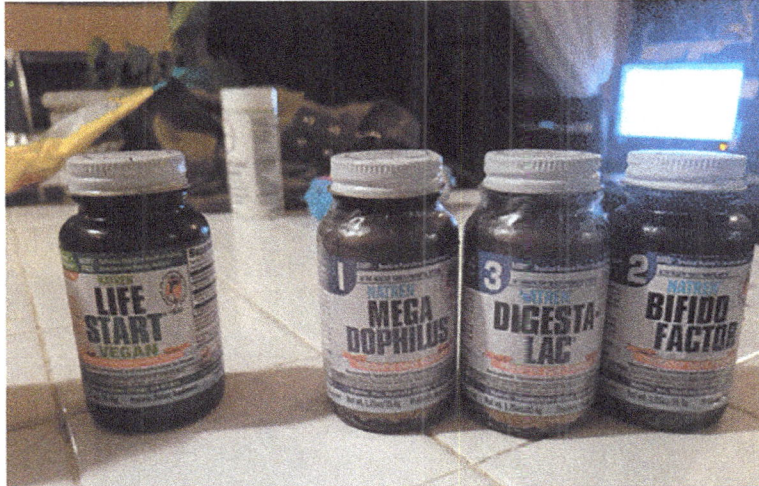

Some of the popular probiotics people take are:

- **Megadophilus** - This is the first step in Natrin's three-step custom probiotic system. This Lactobacillus acidophilus probiotic provides support to the small intestine. Usually where the inflammation is bad.
- **Bifido Factore** - Step 2 in Natrin's three-step program to aid digestion naturally. This is the large intestines now. It's the waist and disposal system.
- **Digesta-Lac** - Step 3 in the program. This Lactobacillus bulgaricus provides support to the large intestines.
- **Enzymes** - We all lack enzymes because pesticides and antibiotics kill these types of good bugs. Enzymes are bugs that live in our food. When we cook our food, we are killing them. They help break down the food that was not able to be broken down. They will enhance your immune system. When you have good digestion, your body can destroy harmful organisms naturally present in food. Enzymes will unlock the energy in food to be broken down to produce energy. Plant-based digestive enzymes have the nutrients necessary for our bodies to maximize the digestion of fruits and veggies. Vitamins do not deliver energy by themselves. They require enzymes for energy. They are vital to metabolism and food digestion. They help us digest, absorb, and utilize nutrients while delivering oxygen throughout the body. These molecules are in all living things. Enzymes control biochemical reactions, including the breakdown of food. Blanching, cooking, processing food, and refrigerating slow down or stop enzyme activity.

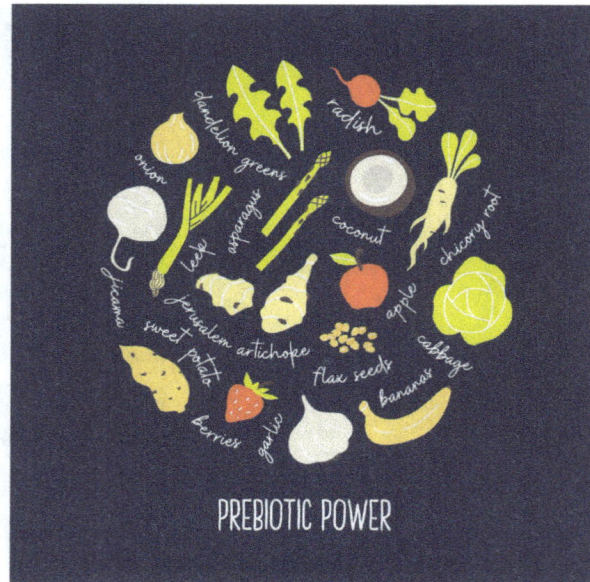

PREBIOTIC POWER

3 Different Sources of Digestive Enzymes:

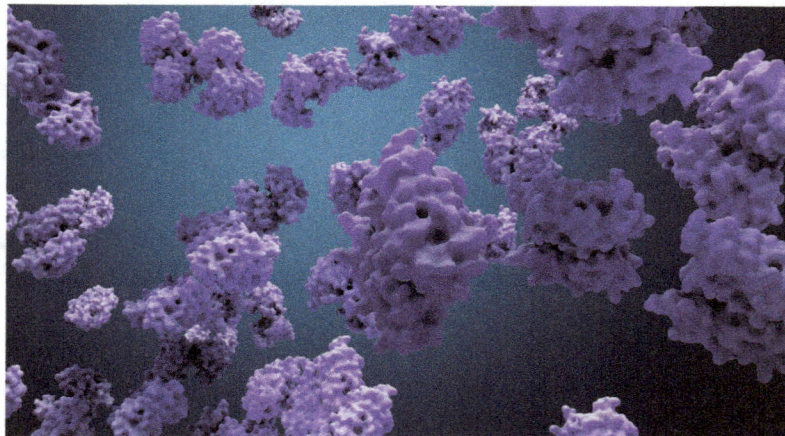

1. Metabolic Enzymes

It lives throughout our entire body system, our organs, bones, blood, and cells. Their job is to grow new cells to maintain the tissue in our bodies.

2. Digestive Enzymes

They are secreted by our various body organs, saliva, stomach, pancreas, and small intestines. They help us digest our foods.

3. Food Enzymes

Exist naturally in the raw food that we consume. It acts like digestive enzymes. You can drink a glass of pineapple juice after consuming large amounts of meat, and it will digest it. After you consume a fruit that has enzymes, like pineapple, and you get that prickly feeling in your mouth, it's actually eating you.

This is caused by proteases. Don`t worry. It`s doing what it`s supposed to do.

Enzymes Diversity:

1. **Proteases** break down proteins.
2. **Lipase** breaks down fats.
3. **Carbohydrase's** such as amylase, which breaks down carbohydrates.
4. **Cellulase** breaks down fiber.
5. **Amylase** breaks down starch.
6. **Lactase** breaks down dairy.
7. **Sucrase** breaks down sugar.
8. **Maltase** breaks down sugar and grains.
9. **Invertase** breaks down sucrose found in cane or beet sugar.
10. **Alph-galactosidase** breaks down starches in beans and cruciferous vegetables.

These enzymes will help get your blood flowing. Your blood will get stagnant or slow-moving when you eat harmful foods and not enough enzymes from fruit.

After a prolonged period and not replenishing them quickly, two things will happen:

1. Your body will work overtime to produce more enzymes, causing the food to be undigested. It will cause stress and, in return, give you inflammation and affects the immune system. It makes it harder to fight diseases.
2. Digestive system eventually slows down, causing food to be undigested. This food stays in your system and ferments and will pollute it. It's then called Toxemia.

Now you can take 2-4 tablespoons of Briggs Apple Cider vinegar. It will provide you with nutrients, enzymes, and probiotics. Everything is necessary to strengthen your immune system. When you are sick, you need extra help through nutrients and probiotics.

A good way to absorb these enzymes is by taking a shot of lemon or orange juice with them. The raw juice provides oxygen and hydrogen into the blood. It's essential for your body to heal.

Juice with labeling on it that reads "not from concentrate" means no water has been added and has not been reconstituted in any way. Concentrated means juice is squeezed and stored in big vats. They start removing oxygen to allow the liquid to keep for up to a year without spoiling, and water is then added when ready to use.

Fragrant companies are hired to create these flavor packs to taste like juice. Any taste difference in drinks like Minute made and Tropicana is from specific flavor packs. Since the flavor packets are made from orange by-products, they don't have to be considered an ingredient and therefore are not required to be on food labels. This is despite the fact they are chemically altered. Hopefully, this helps you to choose a good juice or to pull out your juicer. Please don't think you are saving money by getting a deal. These are fake stuff that companies are making money from, don't support it.

Now that I found the secret to a clean gut, I have to help heal my body.

The brain thrives when it`s nourished with essential fatty acids (omega 3s).

DHA is the most abundant fat in the brain. You can get a lot of this from cold wild fish. Choose wild, cold-water fish like Sockeye salmon or Sardines. Farmed raised fish are good to help repopulate the wild fish but lose nutrients, and farmers have to add nutrients to these fish. Fish that have gills help filter out toxins and make the fish lower in acid.

The bottom feeders like Tilapia are the worst for you. It makes your body so acidic and causes inflammation and possible cancer.

Eating this good fat will help vitamins absorb better. When you have chronic diseases, this process can be impaired or if you consume too many omega-6 fatty acids (Canola, palm, soybean, and safflower oil) that are not good for you. You will need vitamins and minerals to absorb these good fats and essential amino acids that our bodies cannot absorb.

- · Vitamin B12
- · Thiamine
- · Folate
- · Vitamin B6
- · Antioxidants

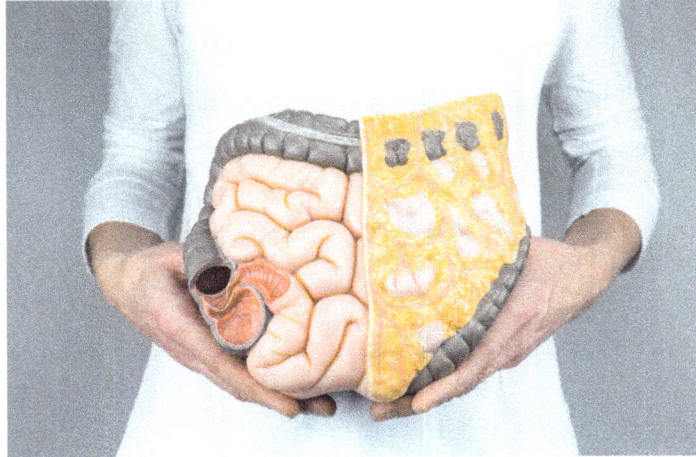

I would love for us all to get these from whole foods, but you need supplements on top of whole foods when you're sick. Scientists are now discovering that your gut will affect your brain health and is linked to depression and gut inflammation.

Your body tells you when your brain is under attack by:

- · Bloating
- · Gas
- · Pain
- · Heartburn
- · Diarrhea
- · Constipation
- · Food sensitivities

Your immune system is attacking you when this happens. You may think these are normal to have, but they are warning signs. When I get a pain in my stomach that feels like knives inside of me trying to get out, that's my red flag to throw down: omega-3 fish oil and enzymes with lemon juice. That's my recipe for stomach issues, and it works like a charm.

There are different ways your brain can become inflamed. One of the main ways doesn't even start in your brain. It starts in your gut. You never even know it. Just like your brain, the inner mucosal lining of your gut has no pain fibers, so even though health issues may start in your gut, it will not tell you there's a problem.

How The Body Is Wired:

Some nerves are under our conscious control while the other is automatic.

The **somatic division** is concerned with voluntary movement—actions we make and control by choice (like intimate feelings and finger movements).

The **Enteric division** controls most of the abdominal organs, mostly the GI tract (stomach and intestines) and, to some extent, the urinary system. These are controlled by automatic control, without stimulation from the brain. Contractions of the muscles in the tract walls must be coordinated carefully to move the digested food along the tract.

When I would having brain fog, I was having gut issues and needed to fix my adrenal glands. That was my body telling me something was wrong.

Now let`s look at the signs of my gut and brain trying to tell me:

PROBLEM	WHERE	SYMPTOM
• not sleeping	brain	when you are confused or cranky in the morning
• stress	brain	not able to speak or think properly, anxiety, anger.
• hormone changes	brain	sad, hair not growing, depressed, anxiety, and anger.
• poor diet	gut	upset stomach, acne, diarrhea, throwing up all the time.
• eating sugar	gut	causes fat, high insulin, sugar highs, and fatigue.
• low omega 3`s	brain	inflammation, pain, diarrhea and brain fog
• gut issues	gut	inflammation, pain, diarrhea
• poor blood flow	brain	not able to breathe good and brain fog.

These are only a few signs that I had. I want you to understand little signs can be something. Once you learn it, then you can make changes to your body and start to heal.

How I helped my adrenal gland and nutrients deficiency was:

- Meditation sounds to get deep sleep (free online).
- Magnesium citrate, calcium, and citrate liquid.
- Serotonin/melatonin- Happy and sleep.
- Amino acid l-glutamine Gama- calming.
- Vitamin A, C, B-1, B-2, B-6, B-12, b-5, Biotin, Folic Acid, Zinc and Copper (food-based formula vitamin Rainbow Light is a vitamin with all this in it together.)
- Chlorophyll - keeps my body alkaline so it can heal.
- Iodine- help hormone (make sure you need it).
- Lots of water and electrolytes to hydrate me and keep things flowing.

Meditation sounds have effects on binaural beats in which the brain entails the hertz difference between different tones played in each ear, focusing the brain on changing its brainwave. This one helped me the most to heal with the binaural beats. I had extreme anxiety, which caused me to have a chronic illness. Calming my mind and using the right nutrients helped my adrenal glands to heal me.

This may seem like a lot, but I only had to take this for a few months or until you feel better.

CHAPTER 5

Look around you! How your environment can hurt or help you

I had to learn how to cook healthy, But the challenge was to learn science and cooking abilities.

Science plays a great deal in the food we eat. Remember, everyone is different, and you can make your own list by using the wellness program in Ch.6. As always, I suggest you work with your primary doctor, nutritionist, or dietitian. You don't realize that you need certain foods to help the other food absorb or emulsify. Now we have been told fat is not good for you. True if you're eating fake hydronated fats like canola oil.

As soon as I cut out this oil from my diet, I was moving again and feeling great. But we need good fats in animals and plants. This fat will give you nutrients like amino acids to help your pituitary glands and adrenal glands.

Monosaturated Fats

Fat molecules have one unsaturated carbon bond in the molecule, which is also called a double bond. Oils that contain monounsaturated fats are typically liquid at room temperature but start to turn solid when cold. Olive oil is an example of a type of oil that contains monounsaturated fats.

A few of my favorite easy digestible healthy fats that I cook with are:

- Pure olive oils (low temperatures)
- Extra virgin coconut oil (high temperatures are ok)
- Grass-fed organic butter
- Ghee (lactose-free)
- Duck fat
- Bacon fat
- Other animal fats
- Avocado oil

These are essential for our body, and we need one of these fats in each meal a day to stay healthy. You can cook with these oils at high temperatures, but the olive oil needs to be cold. If these or any oils start to smoke at any time, you have cooked it too high, making it unhealthy, so toss it out and start over. Oils shelf life is six months and needs to be tossed after.

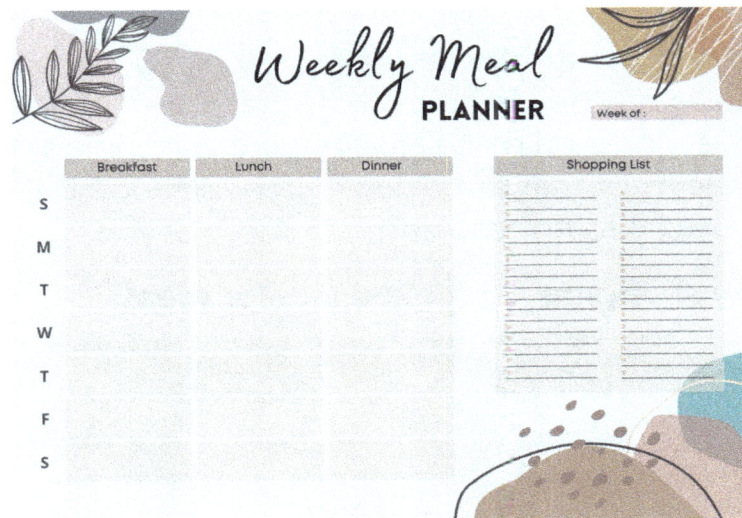

Prepping Your Food

When choosing what to eat and how much, you can hold your hand in a fist, and that would be the size of meat your body needs. Just because it`s on your plate doesn`t mean you should eat it all. Also, your veggies should be 90% and the rest meat. When you look at your plate, you should see way more veggies on it.

Make sure when you look at your plate, the food should not be fake food. It needs to be a whole plant or animal. Think of paleo diets (caveman) and what they consist of. When learning to cook, you want to start out basic and easy for you. Some people go way overboard. They then get frustrated, confused, and give up. I learned how to prep my food all in one day for a month.

Here's What I Did:

Dollar tree/or 99 cent stores

- 30 aluminum containers for the oven.
- 2 boxes of freezer bags
- 30 plastic freezer containers

You may need to go to two different stores to buy all your food. I would go to 99 cent store to get the small stuff and then Costco on the big stuff. Trust me, I have seen people spend $300 and walk out of Costco with two boxes and saying, "What the heck did I buy?." I have lived a very poor life and gained skills from it. I can have a family of three that would live off $100 a month and make great meals.

You may have to go to two stores to buy all your food. Order online helps with impulse buying, go on a full stomach, and make a list and stick to it. You will save a lot from that. I always went shopping on a Sunday and cooked a lot of the meat that same day. Four hours total, but I have all week to be lazy because I was not cooking.

This is what my shopping list looked like for meat:

- 4 whole chickens
- 4 big tri-tips
- 8 lbs Ground beef
- 8 packs of bacon
- 4 cartons of grass-fed eggs

I chose these organic, grass-fed meats, but you can get what you like in large quantities. I would buy from ButcherBox as they save me money with great deals. You can cook half of these meats and freeze them to last even longer.

This is what my list looked like for sides:

- Gluten-free rice
- Gluten-free beans
- Gluten-free noodles
- Gluten-free corn/flour Tortilla shells
- Grass-fed butter or ghee butter

The gluten free was easier to digest for GI problems. Now my organic veggies I chose are:

- Apples
- Oranges
- Lots of lemons
- Grapes
- Arugula salad (lots of vitamins, as an iceberg, has very little)
- Bock Choy
- Potatoes, yams (root veggies have more nutrients in them than above-ground veggies.)
- Lots of frozen veggies. (most frozen veggies are flash-frozen and don't have preservatives on them.)
- Carrots
- Onions
- Garlic
- Green beans

Putting It Together

1. Now, choose seven easy meals with these ingredients.
2. Cook all your meats at one time.
3. Let them cool and then shred the meat. It makes it last longer.
4. Put it all together in your favorite recipe.
5. Throw them in the freezer.
6. When ready to eat, take one out and cook it in the oven.

Save the animal fat in a mason jar with a lid. Use later for cooking. Lots of nutrients there too.

Some days, you like to use a crockpot, then cook the whole chicken and plan to freeze the rest or eat it the next day. Plan on eating chicken and salad one day, then make rolled tacos the next and third day make chicken soup with the left-over chicken and broth.

I could make meals like:

- Lettuce wrap hamburger
- Tacos-chicken, steak, and potato
- Chicken, veggie, potato, and bean soup
- Spaghetti- beef or veggie
- Burritos- egg, chicken, or steak

Substituting Alternatives:

- Milk with plain nut milk, kefir.
- Sugar with honey, molasses,
- Or top with cheese-free sauce.

Now broth is very nutritional for you. It's one of my favorite superfoods as it has wonderful amino acids in it.

Here's a broth recipe that you should have if you are ever sick or on a liquid diet:

- Organic grass-fed chicken
- Carrots
- Garlic
- Celery
- Gray sea salt
- Pepper
- Cayenne pepper
- Water
- Turmeric

Cook in the crockpot for three days on low. Discard the meat and drink the broth. What it does is it cooks the minerals from the bone out, and you get healthy minerals to cure that cold or upset stomach.

Here are some favorite medical recipes I like:

- **Healing Acne** - Manuka Honey is amazing as an antibiotic for the body. Use a UMF grade between 10 and 25. When you are sick, use a higher grade. You can cut the honey down to once a day. Just don't use it with the probiotics, as the honey will kill them. I also take one (1) tablespoon three (3) times a day when I'm sick or have an infection. This stuff saved me from my urethra fistula. Use it topically and eat it. It will heal you. It's also low in glycemic, and diabetics have used it. But check with your doctor. You will lose weight in two weeks by using this stuff. I lost 10 pounds. It gave me energy, and I replaced my sugar with this stuff. Remember, it's a natural food; it's not going to hurt you unless you're one of those rare cases or allergic to bees.

- **Yeast Infections** -You can also use garlic for an antibiotic or pull germs out. You can insert one in and leave overnight, and it will clear up the yeast infection. Also, eat one, and it will help the inside of your gut. Garlic will boost the immune system by producing T-cells that protect our bodies. Eating garlic seems to boost blood cells anti-cancer action. A study found animals that were injected with cancer cells and ate garlic in their food did not develop cancer. An electro biologist discovered that garlic emits a type of ultraviolet radiation known as meta genetic radiation. It is said to stimulate cell growth and activity and have a rejuvenating effect on all body functions.

- **Foods that make you poop** - Don't use if you are the opposite. Make sure to drink 64 oz. of water a day or at least two (2) big cups. Fresh fruit from the berry family, prunes, apples, apricots, beans, and veggies. (Be careful not to eat if you have a fistula or polyps, which can get stuck in your stomach and hurt you.) You can mix flaxseed, psyllium, magnesium, and bentonite clay together and drink one cup at night. In the morning, it will cleanse all the toxins and help you.

- **To relieve a headache** - You can eat organic dark chocolate and caffeine and sit in the bathtub. The chocolate is antibacterial, the body rehydrates you in the bath (usually the case), and caffeine circulates the blood

- **Clams beat Ibuprofen** - Taking glucosamine sulfate, a product derived from shellfish, helps with the pain unless you are allergic don't use.

- **Constipation** - one (1) selenium, one (1) zinc, one (1) tyrosine, four (4) drops of magnesium in water, and four (4) drops of iodine or seaweed.

- **Fistulas** - Wild Oregano oil Mediterranean p-73 Start off with one drop of oregano oil and four (4) drops of olive oil. Put inside your body from down below three (3) times a day. The oregano oil tastes hot like pepper and will burn a little down there. So, go slowly at it. It should help heal the fistula in 2 months or so. This stuff is also used to remove small moles and has been known to help with herpes.
- **Inflammation, pyostomatitis use** Turmeric, pepper, cinnamon, and honey as hot tea.
- **Braggs Nutritional seasoning** - Yeast is a family of fungi family as are mushrooms. Yeast is as nutritional as fruits and vegetables. It has high protein, vitamins, and minerals. Use it in shakes or food. Some people use it instead of cheese. It tastes like in between wheat and cheese. It has health benefits for immune response and anti-cancer properties.

Mamanatural.com has a great recipe for making your own calcium minerals.

You Will Need:

- 1 stockpot
- 1 coffee grinder
- 1 small mason jar with a secure lid
- Organic, grass-fed eggs
- When all done with the eggs, save shells in the carton and keep them in the fridge.
- When you have a dozen, rinse them well in water.
- Fill a stockpot with 6 cups of filtered water and bring to a boil.
- Put the shells in hot water to kill the pathogens.
- Let it cool for 10 minutes. Drain the shells.
- Spread the shells on a glass or stainless-steel baking sheet and let dry overnight. In the morning, put in a 200-degree oven for about 10 minutes to completely dry out.
- Crush shells in a coffee grinder and run until pulverized into a granular form.
- Store in a tightly sealed mason jar away from heat or moisture.

To consume:

1 tsp. contains approximately 800-1,00 mg. of calcium. Consume by mixing ¾ to 1 tsp. daily, divided into three (3) servings with meals. Don`t consume more than 1 tsp. a day as it can irritate sensitive stomachs.

Calcium is the most abundant mineral in our body. It is important for muscle contraction, nerve health, enzyme activity, and cell formation.

Get someone to help you through this journey.

I would like to thank my daughter Barissa for being there when I was in pain or needed a good cheering up. There would be times where I was so sick that my temperature would go so high I would blackout. When she was five, she would help me like she was my nurse. If I didn`t have her to help then, things could have been worse.

I know she has learned a lot from this and had to grow up very quickly. I am so glad to have her in my life. You are the best daughter that anyone could ever have**. I love you for that**.

If you are ever alone and need help, there are meet-up groups with people that have the same chronic conditions. You can meet people who will help you, and you can help them. These people want to meet you too. So please don`t let depression get you. Meetup.com is a great site to look for friends.

Stuff I Used For My Pain:

- *Baths with Epson salt or gray sea salt in it. The salt has minerals in it to help us heal.*
- *Heating and cold pads help ease the pain. When you switch back and forth, your muscle will contract and release the tension. It will circulate the blood flow.*
- *Stomach massage will release stress can encourage intestinal function.*
- *Put castor oil on a piece of flannel and leave it for 1 hour, and it will help the lymph and liver function. The T-cells will boost the body to help specific defense status.*
- *Electrode machine is a low voltage electrical current that stimulates the nerves, and this was my pain reliever.*
- *Pain lotion mixed with peppermint oil, eucalyptus oil, and cannabis oil help with the inflammation. The CBD oil helps make the pain receptors hyperactive, causing them to get hot, desensitizing them, and bringing down the pain-sensing nerve endings.*
- *Peppermint oil pill will help digestion and the spasms in your stomach and relieves the pain.*
- *Pure peanut oil helps with arthritis, joint pain, constipation, and skin disorders. Rub the oil on your skin as it absorbs the monosaturated good oils, which helps prevent heart disease. It has vitamin E to help fight aging free radicals.*

CHAPTER 6

Start Your Journey Now!
Walk of A Wellness Program.

The easy step by step program to your journey of healing in 90 days.

MONTH 1
Week 1

- Make a list of what could be wrong.
- Sign up for a health coach to help you through this process (gutpaincoach.com).
- Check your heart rate, oxygen, measure your muscle activity (download
- apps).
- Check your face maps, Bristol, urine, alkaline test.
- Go to EverlyWell.com and choose all the tests you need to do.
- Iridology
- Decide if you have stress/anxiety and what levels you are at.

Week 2

- Put everything together to find out what is wrong.
- Choose a diet plan that is right for you.
- Make a food journal of foods that you eat and if they hurt you.
- Watch videos on your illness to learn about it.
- Watch videos about real food and fake food.
- Watch videos about sugar and insulin.

Week 3

- Watch the video on fasting and how it can heal you.
- Start your probiotics, enzymes, and prebiotics.
- Bristol/Hydration (charts)

- Have a health coach show you what's inside your body, where your pain is, and what is going to heal it.
- Order an app or have your coach set up a calendar to remind you what to do.
- Use a coach to teach you how to prep your food for the month to stay healthy.
- Get your shopping list set up for a liquid/soft foods diet or set up a delivery for you.

Week 4

- Get your shopping list of Vitamins, Minerals, Trace Minerals, and Amino Acids for you to get or set up a delivery for you.
- Show you quick and easy recipes to be on a liquid/soft food diet and not starve.
- Dump all your bad food from cupboards and buy new healthy foods.
- Talk to your coach about what's inside your food pantry and the environment around you that could be hurting you and clean it up.
- Set up a food delivery service to order healthy food.
- Watch videos on how to cook healthy foods.

MONTH 2
Week 1

- Download an app to track your micronutrients (Myfitnesspal).
- Download An app for brain health (Lumosity).
- Download an app for meditation/ Binaural beats, which helps with stress and anxiety.
- Write in a journal of things that you are grateful for.
- Buy an Omron composition monitor, which is a scale to monitor body muscle and fat.
- Monitor your muscle strength and improve it.

Week 2

- Learn four different healthy meals and implement them in your diet.
- Watch a video on good healthy fats and add them to your diet.
- Youtube HIT workouts and do the quick, short exercises.
- If your stress and anxiety are still high, go to a hypnotist to help with relieving them.
- Order all vitamins, minerals, and nutrients that your body needs.
- Get electrolytes or coconut water to hydrate your body.

Week 3

- Eliminate all bad oils that you cook with and switch to better oils for you.
- Monitor your range of motion by stretching or doing yoga.
- Go over all your health apps and make sure you're improving your health.
- Do a Gut Microbiome test with Everlywell.com.

- Watch a video on healing gut issues with oregano oil, manuka honey, or tea tree oil.
- Check with your coach on your healing.

Week 4

- Learn how to read ingredients and choose the right foods.
- Watch a video on fasting once a month and what it does to your body.
- Learn how to do mindfulness and implement it in your life.
- Learn biofeedback and implement it in your life.
- Check your Bristol chart and learn stomach massage techniques to help be regular.
- Learn how to exercise with pain from Dr. Joe Tatta, google his youtube video.

MONTH 3
Week 1

- Check your Blood pressure and oxygen and check to see if it has gotten better.
- Check to make sure the food you are eating is working for you.
- Check your probiotics and make sure you're taking all three (3) for six months or more.
- Check your inflammation levels from everlywell.com.
- Check your sleep through a sleep pattern device.
- Using a coach has platforms that will monitor your eating, Nutrients, and health to see your improvement visually.

Week 2

- Check your muscle strength and try to improve it.
- Find a purpose in life and implement it.
- Make sure you're taking the right vitamins and not overdoing them.
- Make sure the diet is working for you.
- Check to make sure your depression has gone away through the mindfulness app
- Up your workouts to be more challenging.

Week 3

- Check with a medical advocate that works for you, not the hospital, to help with your insurance bills.
- Watch a video on how to understand your health insurance better.
- Learn ASMR and use it to sleep.
- Manage your emotional stress.
- Go through your food journal to see what is working for you.
- Make sure you can do this on your own.

Week 4

- Try to add four new recipes to your diet.
- Watch a video about training your brain not to feel pain.
- Make your own choices about your body.
- Always think happy thoughts and never negative thoughts.
- Live a pain-free life.

CHAPTER 7

You Cracked the Chronic Illness Code! Now what?

Chronic diseases are the leading cause of death and disability in the United States. Crohn's, Colitis, heart disease, stroke, cancer, type 2 diabetes, and arthritis are just a few chronic diseases. All the medical insurances and billing with chronic illnesses are very confusing, and at times we just ignored it and dealt with what the insurance companies wanted.

It would be best if you always considered getting a medical billing advocate for patients. Be careful of billing advocates that do come to you. They usually work for hospitals, doctors, or pharmacies as they will help you but will go towards who pays their bills. They are not usually for you, so when you look for one, choose advocates for patients. The others will trick you as it has happened to me. Patient advocates that work for you will usually take payment from what you owe, like 20% or 30%. Now, as I do this job myself, it is the hardest job to do. Very confusing as this medical information is all like it's coded in a weird language. Even us billers get very confused. I have done billing for over eight years.

I still have hard times getting doctors, pharmacies, or insurances to approve chronic illness medicines to give to us even when we are in dying need. I had this happen to me. I was on medication, and I had a hospital doctor look at me and my colonoscopy records and approve me to take Humira. Now the whole week, I was in the hospital, and even after, I was not able to get that medicine or even pain medicine. Now I was in the most pain I could even imagine. I kept calling the doctors, the insurance companies, and the pharmacies, and they kept blaming the other person.

I called the ambassadors, Health and Human rights, and nothing for a whole year.

I should have got the medicine. The reason I didn't get the medicine was that I switched insurance and got a new doctor. My old doctor approved it, but the new doctor wanted me to pay him to do another colonoscopy, then he would approve my medicine. This process would take at least two months to do. Then when it goes to the pharmacy, it gets denied because of how much it cost, and my medical wants to deny it. I got added to my fiances Aetna insurance, and the next day they approved my medicine because that insurance was not low-income. Just because you have medical doesn't mean you'll get it. When medication costs over 5,000 a month, you better bet that you won't get it. It cost too much money for them.

Now, to me, it seems that someone was playing a game and wanted to get paid first before my needs.

www.cahealthadvocates.org will help you get the best treatments and lowest payments or toll-free hotline 1800-434-0222.

You want to make sure when you're treating yourself to look at all the different options of other possible problems. You may be diagnosed with Crohn's, and it could be something else. That happened to an estimated 12 million Americans a year.

Misdiagnosis can have serious consequences on a person's health. They can delay recovery or call for harmful treatment. Approximately 40,500 people enter an intensive unit in one year, and a misdiagnosis will cost them their lives. Some of these tests that doctors use are difficult to diagnose because there is no real test to prove their existence. Doctors must play the elimination game too. A patient should have symptoms with Crohn's for at least six months before being seen for a formal evaluation.

With pain, it should be three days a month in the last three months. With other disorders, they can vary. All I'm saying is don't rush into doing surgery until you consider it. In this book, there are ways of looking for the right choice for you to make. It is not a quick fix. Start your path by doing a test, keep your body cleansed of bad chemicals, eat real foods, last educate yourself on your body to be able to make choices.

Knowing that you're in charge of your body will make you strong but also your mind too. Remember, good health is where you need to be.

You will be faced with having to make changes and come up with every excuse for not doing so. You can`t live like this. It will catch up to you. Don`t let these companies make a profit off you. The hardest part is now behind you. Start by doing your 90-day program or working with a coach. (Gutpaincoach.com) You have it way easier than I did. I have all the tools and cheat sheets already done for you. When you get an experienced person to help, you will see things change like you never even thought. When you do not believe in yourself, remember how far your journey has come. Remember everything you have gone through, all the challenges you have succeeded in, and all the pain you have concurred.

Just because your bodies in pain doesn`t mean you can`t change it. I have seen people discover new things to help themselves. You can`t sit around and deal with it just because they tell you can`t. It should give you all the power needed to prove them wrong.

I know this transformation is very painful, and you`re not permanently damaged; you`re just being challenged to be better with a new mind and body so you can be the strongest that you can be.

ALMOND MILK

You`ll Need:

- 1 cup of organic almonds
- 4 cups of water
- A pinch of sea salt

Then:

1. Soak almonds overnight in water and ½ tsp of salt to break down and make beneficial enzymes in the almonds.

2. Blend in the blender and or use a nut juicing bag.

3. Put juice in the fridge as it will last two weeks.

4. You can add a little vanilla for taste.

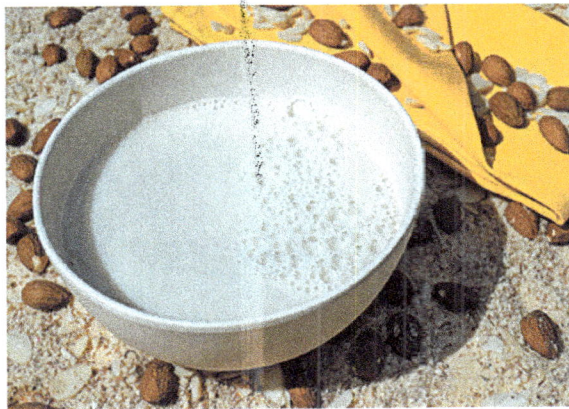

This Photo by Unknown Author is licensed under CC BY-SA

BANANA PANCAKE

You can make a dozen of these and freeze them for later.

- 2 Grass-fed eggs
- 1 banana
- Grass-fed butter or coconut oil
- Mix with egg and banana with a fork until liquid consistency.
- Pour ¼ of the mixture into a hot skillet.
- Let sit until it`s golden and then flip on another side.

It will make four pancakes.

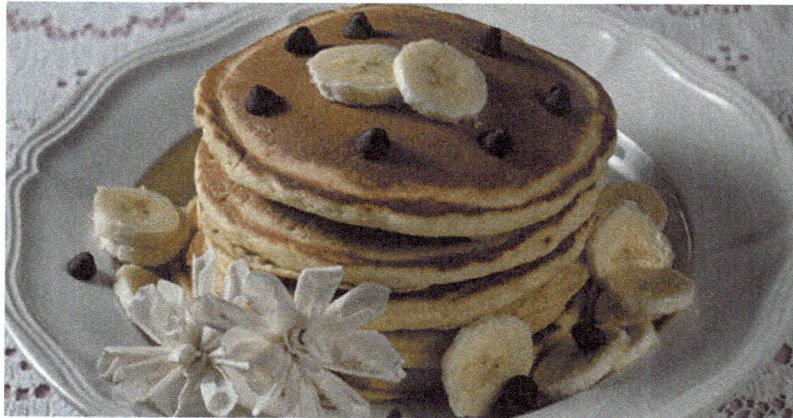

This Photo by Unknown Author is licensed under CC BY

GEROLAMO'S
ESPRESSO GRANITA

You`ll Need:

- · 2 cups espresso/coffee
- · 3 cups of water
- · 3 cups of sugar

Then:

1. Heat on the stove and add the sugar and espresso until blended.
2. Blend in ice maker.
3. Drizzle condensed milk on top.

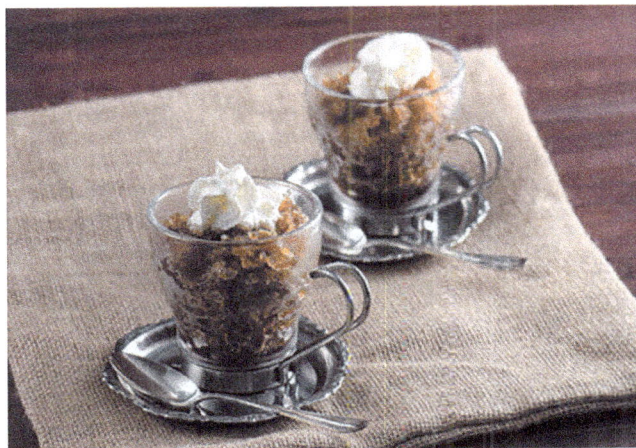

This Photo by Unknown Author is licensed under CC BY-NC-ND

HEALTHY GRANOLA BARS

You`ll Need:

- 2 cups of shredded coconut
- ½ cup of oats
- ½ cup of honey
- ¼ cup of coconut oil melted
- 1 tsp. of pure vanilla
- 1 pinch of salt

To Make:

1. Grease and line a 9x13 baking pan with parchment paper.
2. Combine all ingredients in a food processor.
3. Press the mixture into the lined pan, and smooth on top.
4. Chill one (1) hr. until set and firm.

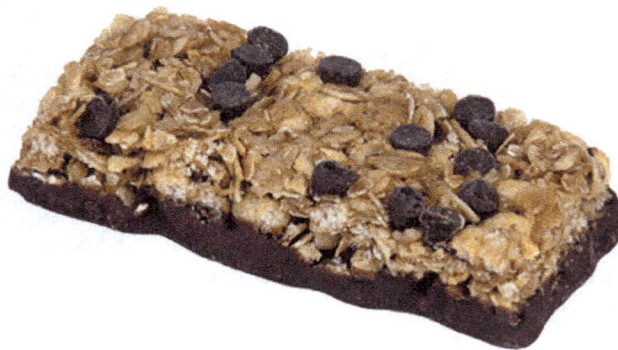

KETO PEANUT BUTTER COOKIES

You`ll Need:

- 1 cup of peanut butter
- 1 egg
- ½ cup of Monk fruit sweetener

To Make:

1. Preheat oven to 350 degrees
2. Combine all ingredients in a bowl.
3. Roll out 15 one inch sized cookie dough balls onto a baking sheet.
4. Use a fork to press down on the tops of the cookie.
5. Bake at 350 degrees for about 10 to 12 minutes.

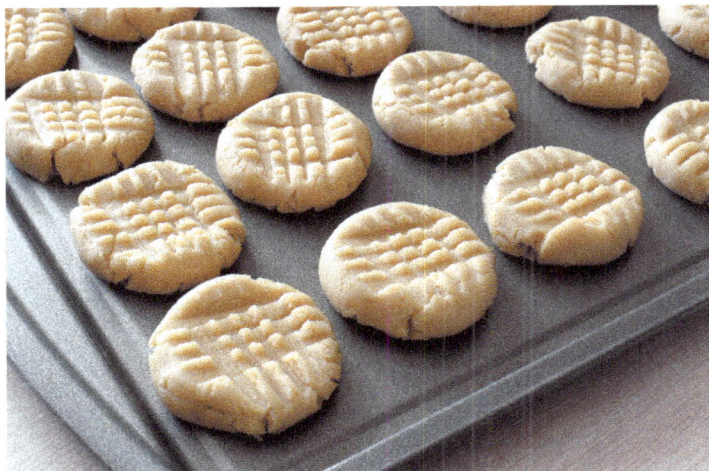

COMPANY CONTACT

Karrie Wilson

San Diego, California

gutpaincoach.com

sdgutpaincoach@gmail.com

(619)993-1662

RESOURCES

Books

Dr. Alice Roberts, The Complete Human Body
Kevin Trudeau, Natural Cures What they don`t want you to know about
Fundamental basis to Iris diagnosis
Jini Patel Thompson, "Listen to Your Gut" listentoyourgut.com
Steven R. Gundry, The Plant Paradox theplantparadox.com
Michael Lenarz, The Chiropractic Way
Products
Bristol chart
Urine acidic test
ASMR
Natrin Probiotics and Enzymes
Brigg`s Vinegar and nutritional yeast

Websites

Cyrex Labs
Ubiodome.com
EvenbetterHealth.com
Dr. Shapiro, mapping
Dr. Mercola Autoimmune Disease
Food and Agriculture organization.com
Livestrong.com

EPILOGUE

I wanted to write this book to show you visually, step by step, to take from the beginning to the end. I noticed many people, including me, would be hesitant to start or give up too easily. I needed a kick in the butt sometimes. Having coaches keeps you motivated. You will get correct information, get healed a lot faster than by yourself. We have parts inside our bodies that need to be taken care of that you didn't know you had to repair. From a person who has been through the same path with chronic illness through my Crohn's disease would help you achieve this.

You wouldn't have to play scavenger hunt to break the chronic code. I would like to show you how I got off my medication and repaired my body without surgery, just by having a better understanding of what was inside my body and why it was so important to fix it.

I do believe that I have cured my disorder, or I have been in remission for almost 17 years now.

We are also getting mixed information that is given to us. When you have a coach, who walked the same path you're walking, gained the experience and knowledge to help you through this terrible time in your life is the easiest way to win this battle.

ABOUT THE AUTHOR

Karrie Wilson is an experienced Chronic Gut Health coach. In her 90 days to pain-free gut and body program, she will show you that every stomach has its issues. She will teach you to find out which bacteria are good to keep in your stomach, also will teach you to know why it's healing you or not, and how she controls her autoimmune disease.

She will meet the client where they are in life and help them figure out where they need to be, and take care of their chronic illness in the easiest way for them. She has learned through experience, which is the best teacher of all time. There are times in your life where you don`t want to let someone else tell you what happens next, and you will get out there and learn it for yourself. You are the only one who will give yourself the best advice.

She went a step further and studied Nutrition, Chronic diseases/disorders, Health, Bacteriology, Eyeology, Anatomy of skin and body, Medical Billing, and Terminology. She will show you how to find things that are not working properly in your body and fix them naturally.

She teaches you to know when you need to go to the doctor and when to wait without hurting your body. With all her visual maps and tools to make the process easy.